QuickFACTS™

From the Experts at the American Cancer Society

Prostate
CANCER

What You Need to Know—NOW

D0840855

Books published by the American Cancer Society

A Breast Cancer Journey: Your Personal Guidebook, Second Edition

American Cancer Society Consumers Guide to Cancer Drugs, Second Edition, Wilkes, Ades, and Krakoff

American Cancer Society's Complete Guide to Colorectal Cancer, Levin et al.

American Cancer Society's Complete Guide to Prostate Cancer, Bostwick et al.

American Cancer Society's Guide to Pain Control, Revised Edition

Angels & Monsters: A child's eye view of cancer, Murray and Howard

Because… Someone I Love Has Cancer: Kids' Activity Book

Cancer in the Family: Helping Children Cope with a Parent's Illness, Heiney et al.

Cancer: What Causes It, What Doesn't

Caregiving: A Step-By-Step Resource for Caring for the Person with Cancer at Home, Revised Edition, Houts and Bucher

Coming to Terms with Cancer: A Glossary of Cancer-Related Terms, Laughlin

Couples Confronting Cancer: Keeping Your Relationship Strong, Fincannon and Bruss

Crossing Divides: A Couple's Story of Cancer, Hope, and Hiking Montana's Continental Divide, Bischke

Eating Well, Staying Well During and After Cancer, Bloch et al.

Good for You! Reducing Your Risk of Developing Cancer

Healthy Me: A Read-along Coloring & Activity Book, Hawthorne (illustrated by Blyth)

Informed Decisions: The Complete Book of Cancer Diagnosis, Treatment, and Recovery, Second Edition, Eyre, Lange, and Morris

Kicking Butts: Quit Smoking and Take Charge of Your Health

Lymphedema: Understanding and Managing Lymphedema After Cancer Treatment

Our Mom Has Cancer, Ackermann and Ackermann

When the Focus Is on Care: Palliative Care and Cancer, Foley et al.

Also by the American Cancer Society

American Cancer Society's Healthy Eating Cookbook: A celebration of food, friends, and healthy living, Third Edition

Celebrate! Healthy Entertaining for Any Occasion

Kids' First Cookbook: Delicious-Nutritious Treats to Make Yourself!

10/06

*Quick*FACTS™

From the Experts at the American Cancer Society

Prostate
CANCER

Published by American Cancer Society / Health Promotions
1599 Clifton Road NE, Atlanta, Georgia 30329, USA

Printed in the United States of America
Cover designed by Jill Dible, Atlanta, GA

5 4 3 2 1   06 07 08 09 10

Library of Congress Cataloging-in-Publication Data
Quick facts prostate cancer : what you need to know—now / from the experts at the American Cancer Society.
     p. cm.
 Includes bibliographical references and index.
 ISBN-13: 978-0-944235-66-9 (pbk. : alk. paper)
 ISBN-10: 0-944235-66-2 (pbk. : alk. paper)
 1. Prostate—Cancer—Popular works. I. American Cancer Society.

 RC280.P7Q53 2007
 616.99'463—dc22

                                        2006016961

A Note to the Reader

This information represents the views of the doctors and nurses serving on the American Cancer Society's Cancer Information Database Editorial Board. These views are based on their interpretation of studies published in medical journals, as well as their own professional experience.

The treatment information in this document is not official policy of the Society and is not intended as medical advice to replace the expertise and judgment of your cancer care team. It is intended to help you and your family make informed decisions, together with your doctor.

Your doctor may have reasons for suggesting a treatment plan different from these general treatment options. Don't hesitate to ask him or her questions about your treatment options.

For more information, contact your American Cancer Society at 800-ACS-2345 or http://www.cancer.org

Table of Contents

Diagnosis and Staging

Treatments and Alternatives

Questions To Ask

Post-Treatment

Latest Research

Resources

Dictionary

Index

Your Prostate Cancer

What Is Cancer?

Cancer* develops when cells in a part of the body begin to grow out of control. Although there are many kinds of cancer, they all start because of out-of-control growth of abnormal cells.

Normal body cells grow, divide, and die in an orderly fashion. During the early years of a person's life, normal cells divide more rapidly until the person becomes an adult. After that, cells in most parts of the body divide only to replace worn-out or dying cells and to repair injuries.

Because cancer cells continue to grow and divide, they are different from normal cells. Instead of dying, they outlive normal cells and continue to form new abnormal cells.

Cancer cells often travel to other parts of the body where they begin to grow and replace normal tissue. This process, called **metastasis**, occurs as the cancer cells get into the bloodstream or lymph vessels of our body. When cells from a cancer like breast cancer spread to another organ like the liver, the cancer is still called breast cancer, not liver cancer.

* Terms in **bold type** are further explained in the dictionary that begins on page 113.

Cancer cells develop because of damage to DNA. This substance is in every cell and directs all its activities. Most of the time when DNA becomes damaged the body is able to repair it. In cancer cells, the damaged DNA is not repaired. People can inherit damaged DNA, which accounts for inherited cancers. Many times, though, a person's DNA becomes damaged by exposure to something in the environment, like smoking.

Cancer usually forms as a **tumor**. Some cancers, like leukemia, do not form tumors. Instead, these cancer cells involve the blood and blood-forming organs and circulate through other tissues where they grow.

Not all tumors are cancerous. **Benign** (non-cancerous) tumors do not spread to other parts of the body (metastasize) and, with very rare exceptions, are not life threatening.

Different types of cancer can behave very differently. For example, lung cancer and breast cancer are very different diseases. They grow at different rates and respond to different treatments. That is why people with cancer need treatment that is aimed at their particular kind of cancer.

Cancer is the second leading cause of death in the United States. Nearly half of all men and a little over one-third of all women in the United States will develop cancer during their lifetimes. Today, millions of people are living with cancer or have had cancer. The risk of developing most types of cancer can be reduced by changes in a person's lifestyle, for example, by quitting smoking and eating a better diet. The sooner a cancer is found and treatment begins, the better are the chances for living for many years.

What Is Prostate Cancer?

About the Prostate

The prostate, found only in men, is a walnut-sized gland located in front of the rectum and underneath the urinary bladder. It contains gland cells that produce some of the seminal fluid, which protects and nourishes sperm cells in semen. Just behind the prostate gland are the seminal vesicles that produce most of the fluid for semen. The prostate surrounds the first part of the urethra, the tube that carries urine from the bladder and semen out of the body through the penis.

Male hormones stimulate the prostate gland to develop in the fetus. Male hormones are also called androgens. The most common androgen is testosterone. The prostate continues to grow as a man reaches adulthood and is maintained after it reaches normal size as long as male hormones are produced. If male hormone levels are low, the prostate gland will not fully develop. In older men, the part of the prostate around the urethra often continues to grow, a condition called **benign prostatic hypertrophy** or **benign prostatic hyperplasia**. This can cause problems with urinating because the overgrowth can narrow the urethral opening.

Although several cell types are found in the prostate, over 99% of prostate cancers develop from the glandular cells. Glandular cells make the seminal fluid that is secreted by the prostate. The medical term for a cancer that starts in glandular cells is **adenocarcinoma**. Because other types of prostate cancer are so rare, if you have prostate cancer, it is almost certain to be an adenocarcinoma.

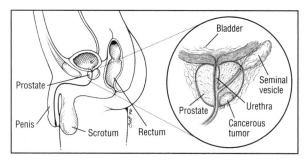

Most prostate cancers grow slowly. Autopsy studies show that many older men who died of other diseases also had prostate cancer that never affected them, and which neither they nor their doctor were aware of. Researchers studying the prostate glands of men who died have found prostate cancer in very few men in their 30s. But this number climbs with age so that by age 80, 70% to 90% of the men will have cancer in their prostate. Some prostate cancers, however, can grow and spread quickly.

Some doctors believe that prostate cancer begins with a condition called **prostatic intraepithelial neoplasia** (PIN). PIN begins to appear in men in their 20s. Almost 50% of men have PIN by the time they reach 50. In this condition, there are changes in the microscopic appearance (size, shape, etc.) of prostate gland cells. These changes are classified as either low grade, meaning they appear almost normal or high grade, meaning they look abnormal.

If you have had high-grade PIN diagnosed on a prostate biopsy, there is a 30% to 50% chance that cancer is also present within your prostate. For this reason, men diagnosed with high-grade PIN are watched carefully and have repeat prostate biopsies.

What Are the Key Statistics About Prostate Cancer?

Prostate cancer is the most common cancer, excluding skin cancers, in American men. The American Cancer Society (ACS) estimates that during 2006 about 234,460 new cases of prostate cancer will be diagnosed in the United States. About 1 man in 6 will be diagnosed with prostate cancer during his lifetime, but only 1 man in 34 in the US population will die of this disease. A little over 1.8 million men in the United States are survivors of prostate cancer.

Prostate cancer is the second leading cause of cancer death in American men, exceeded only by lung cancer. The American Cancer Society estimates that 27,350 men in the United States will die of prostate cancer during 2006. Prostate cancer accounts for about 10% of cancer-related deaths in men.

Ninety one percent of all prostate cancers are found in the local and regional stages (local means it is still confined to the prostate; regional means it has spread from the prostate to nearby areas, but not to distant sites such as bone). The 5-year relative survival rate for these men is nearly 100%.

The 5-year relative survival rate for men whose prostate cancers have already spread to distant parts of the body at the time of diagnosis is about 34%.

Five-year and **10-year survival rates** refer to the percentage of men who live *at least* 5 or 10 years after their prostate cancer is first diagnosed. **Relative survival rates** assumes that people will die of other causes and compare the observed survival with that expected for people without prostate cancer. That means that relative survival only talks about deaths from prostate cancer. Because prostate cancer usually occurs in older men who often have other health problems, relative survival rates are generally used to produce a standard way of discussing prognosis (outlook for survival).

Unfortunately, it is impossible to have completely up-to-date survival figures. To realistically measure 10-year survival rates, we must have records of patients diagnosed at least 13 years ago. We need 10 years of follow-up plus the time it takes to assemble the data.

Modern methods of detection and treatment now mean that prostate cancers are detected earlier and treated more effectively, which has led to a yearly drop in death rate of about 3.5% in recent years. This means that if you are diagnosed this year, your outlook is probably better than the numbers reported above.

Risk Factors and Causes

What Are the Risk Factors for Prostate Cancer?

A **risk factor** is anything that increases your chance of developing a disease such as cancer. Different cancers have different risk factors. For example, exposing skin to strong sunlight is a risk factor for skin cancer. Smoking is a risk factor for cancers of the lungs, mouth, throat, larynx, bladder, and several other organs. But having a risk factor, or even several, does not mean that you will get the disease.

Many people with one or more risk factors never develop cancer, while others with this disease may have no known risk factors. It is important, however, that you know about risk factors so that you can try to change any unhealthy lifestyle behaviors or can choose to have the early detection tests for a potential cancer.

Although we don't yet completely understand the causes of prostate cancer, researchers have found several factors that increase the risk of developing this disease.

Age

The chance of having prostate cancer increases rapidly after age 50. About two-thirds of all prostate cancers are diagnosed in men over the age of 65. It is still unclear why this increase with age occurs.

Race

Prostate cancer occurs about 60% more often in African American men than in white American men. Compared with men of other races, African American men are more likely to be diagnosed at an advanced stage. African American men are more than twice as likely to die of prostate cancer as white men. Prostate cancer occurs less frequently in Asian men than in whites. Hispanic men develop prostate cancer at similar rates as white men. The reasons for these racial differences are not clear.

Nationality

Prostate cancer is most common in North America and northwestern Europe. It is less common in Asia, Africa, Central America, and South America. The reason for this is not well understood, but we know that it is not simply due to better screening in North America and Europe. For example, Chinese men in Los Angeles have one-fifth the prostate cancer rate of white men in the US population.

Family History

Prostate cancer seems to run in some families, suggesting an inherited or genetic factor. Having a father or brother with prostate cancer more than doubles a man's risk of developing this disease. (The risk is higher for men with an affected brother than for those with an affected father.) The risk is much higher for men with several affected relatives, particularly if their relatives were young at the time of diagnosis.

Scientists have identified several inherited genes that seem to increase prostate cancer risk (see next section), but they probably account for only a small fraction of cases. Genetic testing for these genes is not yet available.

Some inherited genes increase risk for more than one type of cancer. For example, inherited mutations of the BRCA1 or BRCA2 genes are the reason that breast and ovarian cancers are much more common in some families. The presence of these gene mutations may also increase prostate cancer risk in some men, but they are responsible for a very small percentage of prostate cancer cases.

Diet

Men who eat a lot of red meat or who have a lot of high-fat dairy products in their diet appear to have a slightly higher chance of developing prostate cancer. These men also tend to eat fewer fruits and vegetables. Doctors are not sure which of these factors is responsible for increasing risk.

Some studies have suggested that men who consume a lot of calcium (through diets or supplements) may have a higher risk of developing advanced prostate cancer. Most studies, however, have not found such a link with the levels of calcium commonly consumed in the average diet, and it's important to note that calcium is known to have other important health benefits.

Exercise

In most studies, exercise has not been shown to reduce prostate cancer risk. A recent study from the Harvard School of Public Health, however, found that men over age 65 who exercise vigorously have a lower rate of prostate cancer.

Vasectomy

Some earlier studies suggested that men who have had a **vasectomy** (minor surgery to make men infertile) may have a slightly increased risk for prostate cancer, but this link has not been consistently found. Among the studies that noticed an increase in risk, some found this risk to be highest in men who were younger than 35 when they had a vasectomy.

Research to resolve this issue is still in progress. However, most recent studies have not found any increased risk among men who have had this operation, and fear of an increased risk of developing prostate cancer should not be a reason to avoid a vasectomy.

Do We Know What Causes Prostate Cancer?

We still do not know exactly what causes prostate cancer. But researchers have found some risk factors and are trying to learn just how these factors cause prostate cells to become cancerous. (Please see the section, "What Are the Risk Factors for Prostate Cancer?")

During the past few years, scientists have made great progress in understanding how certain changes in **DNA** can cause normal prostate cells to grow abnormally and form cancers. DNA is the chemical that carries the instructions for nearly everything our cells do. The reason that you might look like your parents is because they are the source of your DNA.

However, DNA affects more than the way you look. Some genes (parts of your DNA) contain instructions for controlling when cells grow and divide. Certain genes that promote cell growth and division are called

oncogenes. Others that slow down cell division or cause cells to die at the right time are called **tumor suppressor genes**. Cancers can be caused by DNA mutations (defects) that turn on oncogenes or turn off tumor suppressor genes.

Some people are more likely to develop certain types of cancer because of DNA mutations they inherited from a parent. Researchers have discovered inherited DNA changes in certain genes that make some men more likely to get prostate cancer. These genetic changes may cause about 5% to 10% of prostate cancers.

Several genes that are mutated and may be responsible for a man's inherited tendency to develop prostate cancer have been described. The first of these is called **HPC1** (abbreviated from **h**ereditary **p**rostate **c**ancer gene **1**). But there are many other genes described that are mutated and may be responsible for hereditary prostate cancer. None of these is a prominent cause of hereditary prostate cancer, and research on these genes is still preliminary. Genetic tests are not yet available.

As mentioned above, mutations of the BRCA1 or BRCA2 genes greatly increase a woman's risk of developing breast or ovarian cancer. Men with BRCA gene changes may have a slight to moderately increased prostate cancer risk. But BRCA changes are believed to account for only a very small number of prostate cancers.

Most DNA mutations related to prostate cancer develop during a man's life rather than having been inherited before birth. Every time a cell prepares to divide into 2 new cells, it must make a copy of its DNA. This process is not perfect, and sometimes errors occur. Fortunately, cells have repair enzymes that correct mistakes in the DNA. But some errors may slip past (especially if the cells are growing rapidly), leaving the flawed DNA in the new cell.

Exposure to radiation or cancer-causing chemicals may cause DNA mutations in many organs of the body, but these factors have not been proven to be important causes of mutations in prostate cells.

There is evidence that development of prostate cancer is linked to increased levels of certain hormones. High levels of androgens (male hormones, such as testosterone) may contribute to prostate cancer risk in some men.

Some researchers have noted that men with high levels of another hormone, insulin-like growth factor-1 (IGF-1), are more likely to develop prostate cancer. IGF-1 hormone is similar to insulin, but its normal function relates to cell growth, not sugar metabolism. Some studies, however, have not found any associations between IGF-1 and prostate cancer risk. Further research is needed to figure out the practical value of these observations.

Prevention and Detection

Can Prostate Cancer Be Prevented?

Because the exact cause of prostate cancer is not known, at this time it is not possible to prevent most cases of the disease. Many risk factors such as age, race, and family history cannot be controlled.

Current information on prostate cancer risk factors, however, suggests that some cases might be prevented.

Diet

You may be able to reduce your risk of prostate cancer by changing the way you eat.

The American Cancer Society recommends eating a variety of healthful foods, with an emphasis on plant sources, and limiting your intake of red meats, especially those high in fat or processed. Eat 5 or more servings of fruits and vegetables each day. Bread, cereals, grain products, rice, pasta, and beans are also recommended. These guidelines on nutrition may also lower the risk for some other types of cancer, as well as other health problems.

Tomatoes (raw, cooked, or in tomato products such as sauces or ketchup), pink grapefruit, and watermelon are rich in **lycopenes**. These vitamin-like substances are antioxidants that help prevent damage to DNA and may help lower prostate cancer risk.

Taking vitamin or mineral supplements may affect your prostate cancer risk, but this is not yet clear. Some studies suggest that taking 50 milligrams (or 400 International Units) of **vitamin E** daily can lower risk. Other studies have concluded that vitamin E supplements have no impact on cancer risk and may increase risk for some kinds of heart diseases. **Selenium**, a mineral, may also lower risk. On the other hand, vitamin A supplements may actually increase prostate cancer risk. Taking supplements can have risks and benefits and before starting vitamins or other supplements, you should talk with your doctor.

The Selenium and Vitamin E Cancer Prevention Trial (SELECT) is a large clinical trial designed to determine if either (or both) of these 2 supplements can help protect against prostate cancer. The study opened in 2001 and has enrolled more than 32,000 men. The results of the study will probably not be available for several years.

Medications

Some drugs may also help reduce the risk of prostate cancer.

Researchers have been interested in determining whether a drug called finasteride (Proscar), which is already used to treat benign prostatic hyperplasia (BPH), can reduce prostate cancer risk. Finasteride prevents the body from making a certain potent androgen (male hormone). Androgens are known to be important in promoting the growth of normal and cancerous prostate cells and may play a part in the development of prostate cancers.

The Prostate Cancer Prevention Trial (PCPT) was a study that enrolled more than 18,000 men to determine whether finasteride reduced the risk of developing prostate cancer. Each man in the study was randomly assigned to take either finasteride or a placebo pill (sugar pill) each day for 7 years. The men didn't know which pill they were taking.

At the end of the study, the men taking finasteride were about 25% less likely to have developed prostate cancer than those getting the placebo. But the cancers that developed in the men taking finasteride looked like they were more likely to grow and spread. The reason for this is not known. The study researchers are continuing to watch these men to see if these cancers truly are more aggressive.

The men taking finasteride were more likely to experience sexual side effects, such as decreased sexual desire and episodes of impotence, than those taking placebo. But they were less likely to have urinary problems, such as difficulty urinating and inability to hold urine in (incontinence).

At this time, it is unclear if taking finasteride to prevent prostate cancer is a good thing. The results of the PCPT will become clearer over the next few years.

Can Prostate Cancer Be Found Early?

Prostate cancer can often be found early by testing the amount of **prostate-specific antigen** (**PSA**—see pages 16–22) in your blood. Prostate cancer may also be found when your doctor does a **digital rectal exam (DRE)**. Because your prostate gland lies just in front of your rectum, the doctor can feel if there are any nodules or areas of abnormal hardness in your prostate. These indicate the need for further testing to see if there is a cancer. If you have routine yearly exams and either one of these test results becomes abnormal, then any cancer you might have has probably been found at an early, more treatable stage.

Since the use of early detection tests for prostate cancer became relatively common (about 1990), the prostate cancer death rate has dropped. But it has not been proven that this is a direct result of screening.

There are potential problems with the current screening methods. Neither the PSA test nor the DRE is 100% accurate. Inconclusive or false results on testing could cause confusion and anxiety. Some men might have a prostate biopsy (which carries its own small risks along with discomfort) when cancer is not present, while others might get a false sense of security from normal test results when cancer is actually present.

Until more information is available, whether you have the tests is something for you and your doctor to decide. Things to consider are your age and health. If you are young and develop prostate cancer, it will probably shorten your life if it is not caught early. If you are older or in poor health, then prostate cancer may never become a major problem because it is generally a slow-growing cancer.

ACS Recommendations for the Early Detection of Prostate Cancer

The American Cancer Society believes that health care professionals should offer the prostate-specific antigen (PSA) blood test and digital rectal exam (DRE) yearly, beginning at age 50, to men who have at least a 10-year life expectancy. Men at high risk, such as African Americans and men who have a first-degree relative (father, brother, or son) diagnosed with prostate cancer at an early age (younger than age 65), should begin testing at age 45.

Men at even higher risk (because they have several first-degree relatives who had prostate cancer at an early age) could begin testing at age 40. Depending on the results of this initial test, further testing might not be needed until age 45.

Health care professionals should give men the opportunity to openly discuss the benefits and risks of testing at annual checkups. Men should actively participate in the decision by learning about prostate cancer and the pros and cons of early detection and treatment of prostate cancer.

Recommendations of other organizations

No major scientific or medical organizations, including the American Cancer Society (ACS), American Urological Association (AUA), US Preventive Services Task Force (USPSTF), American College of Physicians (ACP), National Cancer Institute (NCI), American Academy of Family Physicians (AAFP), and American College of Preventive Medicine (ACPM) advocate routine testing for prostate cancer at this time. The USPSTF has concluded that studies completed so far do not provide enough evidence to determine whether the benefits of testing for early prostate cancer outweigh the disadvantages.

The ACS, AUA, ACP, NCI, AAFP, and ACPM recommend that health care professionals discuss the option of testing for early detection of prostate cancer with men. They recommend discussing the potential benefits, side effects, and unresolved questions regarding early prostate cancer detection and treatment so that men can make individualized and informed decisions about testing. In addition, the American Cancer Society and the American Urological Association recommend that health care professionals offer the option of testing for early detection of prostate cancer to men who are at least 50 years old (or younger if at higher risk).

Prostate-Specific Antigen (PSA) Blood Test

Prostate-specific antigen (PSA) is a substance made by the normal prostate gland. Although PSA is mostly found in semen, a small amount is also present in the blood. Most men have levels under 4 nanograms per milliliter (ng/mL) of blood.

When prostate cancer develops, the PSA level usually goes above 4. If your level is in the borderline range between 4 and 10, you have about a 25% chance of having prostate cancer. If it is more than 10, your chance of having prostate cancer is over 50% and increases further as your PSA level increases. But it is important to remember that about 15% of men with a PSA below 4 will have prostate cancer on biopsy.

Your PSA level can also be affected by other factors:

- It increases with noncancerous enlargement of the prostate (called benign prostatic hyperplasia, or BPH), something many men have as they grow older.
- It can also increase with **prostatitis**, an infection or inflammation of the prostate gland.
- Your PSA will also normally go up slowly as you *age*, even if you have no prostate abnormality.

- **Ejaculation** can cause a temporary increase in blood PSA levels, so some doctors will suggest that men abstain from ejaculation for 2 days before testing.
- Some *medicines* may affect blood PSA levels. You should tell your doctor if you are taking *finasteride* (Proscar or Propecia) or *dutasteride* (Avodart), as these medicines may falsely lower PSA levels and require the doctor to adjust the reading.
- *Herbal preparations* may also affect blood PSA levels. Herbal mixtures that are dietary supplements marketed "for prostate health" may affect PSA levels. For example, they could potentially mask an elevated PSA level, which is why it is important to let your doctor know if you are taking any type of supplement. Saw palmetto (an herb used by some men to treat BPH) does not seem to interfere with the measurement of PSA.

If your PSA level is high, your doctor may recommend a prostate biopsy (discussed later) to determine if you have cancer. Before doing that, however, there are some new types of PSA tests that might help determine if you need a prostate biopsy.

Not all doctors agree on how to use these additional PSA tests. If your PSA test result is not normal, ask your doctor to discuss your cancer risk and your need for further tests.

Percent-free PSA

PSA occurs in 2 major forms in the blood. One is attached to blood proteins and the other circulates free (unattached). The percent-free PSA test indicates how much PSA circulates free compared to the total PSA level. The percentage of free PSA is lower in men who have prostate cancer than in men who do not.

If your PSA results are in the borderline range (4-10 ng/mL), a low percent-free PSA (less than 10%) means that your likelihood of having prostate cancer is about 50% and that you should probably have a biopsy. In fact, many doctors recommend biopsies for men whose percent-free PSA is 25% or less. A recent study found that if men with borderline PSA results had prostate biopsies only when their percent-free PSA was 25% or less, about 20% of unnecessary prostate biopsies could be avoided, and about 95% of cancers would still be detected. Although this test is widely used, not all doctors agree that 25% is the best "cutoff point" to decide on a biopsy.

PSA velocity

The PSA velocity is not a separate test. It indicates how fast the PSA rises over time. Even when the total PSA value isn't over 4 ng/mL, a high PSA velocity suggests that cancer may be present and a biopsy should be considered. For example, if your PSA was 1.7 on one test, and then a year later was 3.8, that is a rapid rise and cause for concern.

This can be useful if you are having the PSA test every year. If it goes up faster than 0.75 ng/mL per year (for example, if values went from 2 to 2.8 to 3.6 over the course of 2 years), it is considered high, and a biopsy should be considered. Most doctors believe that in order to be valid, the PSA velocity should be measured over a minimum of 18 months.

PSA density

The PSA density (PSAD) is used for men with large prostate glands. The doctor determines the volume of the prostate gland with transrectal ultrasound (discussed below) and divides the PSA number by the prostate volume. A higher PSA density (PSAD) indicates greater likelihood of cancer. PSA density has not been that useful. The percent-free PSA test has thus far been shown to be more accurate.

Age-specific PSA ranges

A PSA result within the borderline range might be very worrisome in a 50-year-old man but cause less concern in an 80-year-old man. It is known that PSA levels are normally higher in older men than in younger men, even in the absence of cancer. For this reason, some doctors have suggested comparing PSA results with results from other men of the same age.

But because the usefulness of age-specific PSA ranges is not well proven, the manufacturers of the PSA tests, most doctors and professional organizations do not recommend their use at this time.

The PSA dilemma

There is no question that the PSA test can help spot prostate cancer. But it can't tell how dangerous the cancer is. The problem is that some prostate cancers are slow growing and may never cause problems. But because of an elevated PSA level, many men will be diagnosed with a prostate cancer that would never lead to their death. Yet they are being treated with either surgery or radiation because they are uncomfortable not having treatment. Doctors and patients are still struggling to decide who should receive treatment and who can be followed without treatment.

Use of the PSA Blood Test After Prostate Cancer Diagnosis

Although the PSA test is used mainly to detect prostate cancer early, it is valuable in other situations:

- The PSA test can be used together with clinical exam results and tumor grade to help decide which tests are needed for further evaluation.
- It can help determine whether your cancer is still confined to the prostate gland. If your PSA level is very high, your cancer has probably spread beyond the prostate. This may affect your treatment options, since some forms of therapy (such as surgery and radiation) are not likely to be helpful if the cancer has spread to the lymph nodes or other organs.
- After surgery or radiation treatment, the PSA level can be monitored to help determine if the treatment were successful. PSA levels normally fall to very low levels if the treatment removed or destroyed all of the prostate cells. A rising PSA level can mean that prostate cancer cells are present and your cancer has come back.
- If you choose a "watchful waiting" approach to treatment, the PSA level can help determine if the disease is progressing and if active treatment should be considered.
- During hormonal therapy or chemotherapy, the PSA level can help indicate how well the treatment is working or when it may be time to try a different form of treatment.

Once prostate cancer has recurred, or if it has spread outside of the prostate (metastatic disease), doctors are not interested in the actual number but instead whether it changes. The PSA number does not predict whether or not a person will have symptoms or how long he will live. The PSA result of 4 that is associated with a normal level is no longer used. Many people have very high PSA values and feel just fine. Other people have low values and have symptoms. With advanced disease, it may be more important to look at the way the PSA level is changing rather than the actual number.

Digital Rectal Exam (DRE)

During this exam, a doctor inserts a gloved, lubricated finger into the rectum to feel for any irregular or firm area that might be a cancer. The prostate gland is located just in front of the rectum, and most cancers begin in the back part of the gland that can be reached by a rectal exam. While it is uncomfortable, the exam causes no pain and only takes a short time.

Although DRE is less effective than the PSA blood test in finding prostate cancer, it can sometimes find cancers in men with normal PSA levels. For this reason, the American Cancer Society guidelines recommend that when prostate cancer screening is done, both the DRE and PSA blood test should be used.

The DRE is also used once a man is known to have prostate cancer to help determine if the cancer has spread beyond his prostate gland and to detect cancer that has come back after treatment.

Transrectal Ultrasound (TRUS)

Transrectal ultrasound (TRUS) uses sound waves to make an image of the prostate on a video screen. When a small probe is placed in the rectum, sound waves enter the prostate and create echoes that are picked up by the probe. A computer turns the pattern of echoes into a picture.

You will feel some pressure when the TRUS probe is placed in your rectum. The procedure takes only a few minutes and is done in a doctor's office or outpatient clinic.

TRUS is usually not recommended as a routine test by itself to detect prostate cancer because it doesn't often spot early cancer. Instead, it is most commonly used during a prostate biopsy (described in the next section). TRUS is used to guide the biopsy needle into exactly the right area of the prostate.

TRUS is useful in other situations as well. It can be used to measure the size of the prostate gland, which can help determine the PSA density and may also affect which treatment options a man has. It is also used as a guide during some forms of treatment, such as **cryosurgery**.

Diagnosis and Staging

How Is Prostate Cancer Diagnosed?

If certain symptoms or the results of early detection tests—the prostate-specific antigen (PSA) blood test and/or digital rectal exam (DRE)—have raised the possibility of prostate cancer, your doctor will do a prostate biopsy to find out if the disease is present.

Signs and Symptoms of Prostate Cancer

Early prostate cancer usually causes no symptoms and is most often found by a PSA test and/or DRE. Some advanced prostate cancers can slow or weaken your urinary stream or make you need to urinate more often. But non-cancerous diseases of the prostate, such as BPH (benign prostatic hyperplasia) are a more common cause of these symptoms.

If the prostate cancer is advanced, you might develop blood in your urine (hematuria) or difficulty getting an erection (impotence). Advanced prostate cancer commonly spreads to the bones, which can cause pain in the hips, spine, ribs, or other areas. Cancer that has spread to the spine can also cause it to press on the spinal nerves, which can result in weakness or numbness in the legs or feet, or even loss of bladder or bowel control.

Other diseases, however, can also cause many of these same symptoms. It is important to tell your doctor about any of them so that the cause can be determined and treated.

The Prostate Biopsy

A **core needle biopsy** is the main method used to diagnose prostate cancer. It is usually done by a urologist, a surgeon who treats cancers of the genitourinary tract, which includes the prostate gland. A biopsy is a procedure in which a sample of tissue is removed and then examined under a microscope. Using transrectal ultrasound to "see" the prostate gland, the doctor quickly inserts a needle through the wall of the rectum into the prostate gland and rapidly removes it. The needle will contain a cylinder of tissue, usually about $1/2$-inch long and $1/16$-inch across. This is repeated from 8 to 18 times, although most urologists will do about 12 biopsies. These are sent to the lab to see if cancer is present.

Though the procedure sounds painful, it typically causes only a very brief, uncomfortable sensation because it is done with a special instrument called a biopsy gun. The biopsy gun inserts and removes the needles in a fraction of a second. Most doctors who do the biopsy will numb the area with local anesthetic. You might want to ask your doctor if he or she will numb the area first with a local anesthetic.

Unfortunately, even when taking many samples, biopsies can still sometimes miss detecting cancer if none of the biopsy needles pass through it. This is known as a "false negative" result. If your doctor still strongly suspects you may have prostate cancer (due to a very high PSA level, for example) a repeat biopsy may be needed to help rule this out.

Some doctors will perform the biopsy through the perineum, the skin between the rectum and the scrotum. The doctor will place his or her finger in your rectum to feel the prostate and then insert the biopsy needle through a small incision in the skin of the perineum. The doctor will also use a local anesthetic to numb the area.

The biopsy procedure itself takes about 15 minutes and is usually done in the doctor's office. You will likely be given antibiotics before the biopsy to reduce the risk of infection. For a few days after the procedure, you may feel some soreness in the area, and will notice blood in your urine and light bleeding from your rectum. Many men also see some blood in their semen for a while after the biopsy.

Your biopsy sample will be sent to a pathology lab. There, the pathologist (a doctor who specializes in diagnosing disease in tissue samples) will determine if there are cancer cells in your biopsy sample by looking at it under the microscope. Getting the results usually takes 1 to 3 days, but it could take longer. If cancer is present, the pathologist will also assign it a **grade**.

Grading the Prostate Cancer

Almost all pathologists grade prostate cancers according to the Gleason system. This system assigns a **Gleason grade**, using numbers from 1 to 5 based on how much the arrangement of cells in the cancerous tissue looks like normal prostate tissue.

- If the cancerous tissue looks much like normal prostate tissue, a grade of 1 is assigned.

- If the cancer lacks these features and its cells seem to be spread haphazardly through the prostate, it is called a grade 5 tumor.
- Grades 2 through 4 have intermediate features.

Because prostate cancers often have areas with different grades, a grade is assigned to the 2 areas that make up most of the cancer. These 2 grades are added together to yield the **Gleason score** (also called the Gleason sum) between 2 and 10. The higher your Gleason score, the more likely it is that your cancer will grow and spread rapidly.

"Suspicious" Results

Sometimes, when the pathologist looks at the prostate cells under the microscope, they don't look cancerous, but they're not quite normal, either. These results are often reported as "suspicious." They generally fall into 2 categories—either atypical or prostatic intraepithelial neoplasia (PIN).

PIN is often divided into low grade and high grade. Many men begin to develop low-grade PIN at an early age and do not necessarily develop prostate cancer. The importance of low-grade PIN in relation to prostate cancer is still unclear.

But with atypical findings or high-grade PIN, cancer may already be present somewhere else in the prostate gland. For high-grade PIN, there is a 30% to 50% chance of finding prostate cancer on a later biopsy. For this reason, repeat prostate biopsies are often recommended in these cases.

How Is Prostate Cancer Staged?

The stage of a cancer is the most important factor in choosing treatment options and predicting a patient's outlook for survival. If your prostate biopsy confirms a cancer, more tests may be done to find out how far the cancer has spread within the prostate, to nearby tissues, or to other parts of the body. This process, called **staging**, gathers information about a cancer from various tests to determine how widespread it is.

Your doctor will use your digital rectal exam (DRE) results, prostate-specific antigen (PSA) level, and Gleason score to determine how likely it is that your cancer has spread outside of the prostate. This information is used to decide which other tests (if any) to order. Men with a normal DRE result, a low PSA, and a low Gleason score may not need any other tests, because the chance that the cancer has spread is so low.

Medical History and Physical Exam

The physical exam, especially the DRE, is an important part of prostate cancer staging. By doing a DRE your doctor can sometimes tell whether the cancer is only on one side of the prostate, whether it is present on both sides, or whether it has probably spread beyond the prostate gland. The DRE is always used together with the PSA blood test for early detection of prostate cancer and is discussed in the section, "Can Prostate Cancer Be Found Early?" (See page 23.)

Your doctor may also examine other areas of your body to see if the cancer has spread outside your pelvis. In addition, your doctor will also ask you about symptoms such as bone pain, which may indicate that the cancer has spread to your bones.

Imaging Tests Used for Prostate Cancer Staging

Not all men with prostate cancer need to have imaging tests, but for those who do, the following tests are sometimes used.

Radionuclide bone scan

When prostate cancer spreads, it commonly goes to the bones first. Even when prostate cancer spreads to the bone, it is still called prostate cancer not bone cancer. A **bone scan** can help show whether cancer has reached the bones.

For this test, a small amount of radioactive material is injected **intravenously** (IV) into the blood. The radioactive substance settles in damaged bone tissue throughout the entire skeleton over the course of a couple of hours. You then lie on a table for about 30 minutes while a special camera detects the radioactivity and creates a picture of your skeleton.

Areas of bone damage appear as "hot spots" in your skeleton—that is, they attract the radioactivity. These areas may suggest metastatic cancer is present, but arthritis or other bone diseases can also cause the same pattern. To distinguish between these conditions, your cancer care team may use other imaging tests such as simple **x-rays** or **CT** or **MRI** scans, or they may even take biopsy samples of the bone.

The injection itself is the only uncomfortable part of the scanning procedure. The radioactive material is passed out of the body in the urine over the next few days. Because the amount of radioactivity used is very low, it carries very little risk to you or others, but you may want to ask your doctor if you should take any special precautions after having this test.

Computed tomography (CT)

The CT scan (also known as a CAT scan) is an x-ray procedure that produces detailed, cross-sectional images of your body. Instead of taking one picture, like a conventional x-ray, a CT scanner takes many pictures of the part of your body being studied as it rotates around you. A computer then combines these pictures into an image of a slice of your body.

This test can help tell if prostate cancer has spread into lymph nodes in your pelvis. If your prostate cancer has come back after treatment, the CT scan can often tell whether it is growing into structures in your pelvis. On the other hand, CT scans rarely provide useful information about newly diagnosed prostate cancers that are believed to be localized (confined to the prostate) based on their clinical stage, PSA level, and Gleason score. CT scans are not as useful as magnetic resonance imaging (MRI) for evaluating the prostate gland itself.

CT scans take longer than regular x-rays. You need to lie still on a table, and the part of your body being examined is placed within the scanner, a doughnut-shaped machine that completely surrounds the table. You might feel a bit confined by the ring you have to lie in when the pictures are being taken.

After the first set of pictures is taken you may be asked to drink 1 or 2 pints of a radiocontrast agent, or "dye." You may also receive an IV (intravenous) line through which the contrast dye is injected. This helps better outline structures in your body. You will also need to drink enough liquid to have a full bladder in order to keep the bowel away from the area of the prostate gland. A second set of pictures is then taken.

The solution you drink and the injection may cause some flushing (a feeling of warmth, especially in the face). Some people are allergic and get hives. Rarely, more serious reactions like trouble breathing or low blood pressure can occur. Be sure to tell the doctor if you have ever had a reaction to any contrast material used for x-rays.

Magnetic resonance imaging (MRI)

MRI scans use radio waves and strong magnets instead of x-rays. The energy from the radio waves is absorbed by the body and then released in a pattern formed by the type of tissue and by certain diseases. A computer translates the pattern of radio waves into a very detailed image of parts of the body. This produces cross-sectional slices of the body like a CT scanner, but it can also show slices (views) from several angles. As with CT scans, a contrast material might be injected, but this is done less often.

MRI scans can be very helpful in looking at prostate cancer. They can produce a very clear picture of the prostate and show whether the cancer has spread outside the prostate into the seminal vesicles or the bladder. This information can be very important for your doctors in planning your treatment.

MRI scans take longer than CT scans—often up to an hour. During the scan, you lie inside a narrow tube, which is confining and can upset people who don't like enclosed spaces. The machine also makes a thumping noise. Some places provide headphones with music to block this out. To improve the accuracy of the MRI, many doctors will place a probe, called an endorectal coil, inside your rectum. This must stay in place for 30 to 45 minutes and can be uncomfortable.

ProstaScint™ scan

Like the bone scan, the **ProstaScint** scan uses an injection of low-level radioactive material to find cancer that has spread beyond the prostate. Both tests look for areas of the body where the radioactive material collects. But there are important differences between the tests.

The radioactive material used for the bone scan is attracted specifically to bone; it collects in areas of bone that may be damaged by prostate cancer, other cancers, or benign conditions. The radioactive material for the ProstaScint scan is attracted specifically to prostate cells in the body. It is attached to a monoclonal antibody, a type of manmade protein that recognizes and sticks to a particular substance. In this case, the antibody specifically sticks to prostate-specific membrane antigen (PSMA), a substance found at high levels in normal and cancerous prostate cells.

The advantage of this test is that it can detect the spread of prostate cancer to lymph nodes and other soft (non-bone) organs and can distinguish prostate cancer from other cancers and benign disorders. But most doctors do not recommend this test for men who have just been diagnosed with prostate cancer. It may be useful if your blood PSA level begins to rise after treatment and other tests are not able to find the exact location of your cancer, but doctors may not order this test if they believe it will not be helpful for a particular patient.

Lymph Node Biopsy

A lymph node biopsy (also called a lymph node dissection) is sometimes done to find out if your cancer has spread from your prostate to nearby lymph nodes. If cancer cells are found in the lymph node biopsy specimen, surgery to cure the cancer is usually not done; other treatment options are considered. Lymph node biopsies are rarely done unless your doctor is concerned that the cancer has spread. There are several ways to biopsy lymph nodes.

Surgical biopsy

The surgeon may remove lymph nodes through an incision in the lower part of your abdomen. This is often done in the same operation as the planned radical prostatectomy (see the section on "How Is Prostate Cancer Treated?" for information about radical prostatectomy).

If the surgeon has a reason to suspect that the cancer may have spread (such as a PSA level over 20 or a Gleason score over 7), he or she may remove the nodes before attempting to remove the prostate gland. A pathologist then examines the nodes while you are still under anesthesia to help the surgeon decide whether to continue the radical prostatectomy. This is called a **frozen section** exam, because the tissue sample is frozen before thin slices are taken to check under a microscope. If the nodes contain cancer, the operation is usually stopped. This is because removing the prostate would be unlikely to cure the cancer, but it could still result in serious complications or side effects.

If the likelihood of spread is low, most surgeons do not request a frozen section exam and instead send the lymph nodes to be examined with the removed prostate gland. The testing results are typically available 3 to 7 days after surgery.

Laparoscopy

A surgeon may use a **laparoscope**—a long, slender tube with a small video camera on the end—inserted into the abdomen through a very small incision. The surgeon removes all of the lymph nodes around the prostate gland using special surgical instruments operated through the laparoscope and sends them to the pathologist. Because there are no large incisions, most people recover fully in only 1 or 2 days, and the operation leaves virtually no scar. This procedure is not common, but it is sometimes used when knowing the lymph node status is important and radical prostatectomy is not planned (such as for certain men who choose treatment with radiation therapy).

Fine needle aspiration (FNA)

If your lymph nodes appear enlarged on an imaging study (CT or MRI) a specially trained radiologist may take a sample of cells from an enlarged lymph node by using a technique called **fine needle aspiration** (FNA). In this procedure, the doctor uses the CT scan image to guide a long, thin needle into an enlarged lymph node. The syringe attached to the needle takes a small tissue sample from the node. Before the needle is placed, your skin will be numbed with local anesthesia. You will be able to return home a few hours after the procedure. This procedure is not used very often.

The TNM Staging System

A staging system is a standardized way in which the cancer care team describes the extent to which a cancer has spread. While there are several different staging systems for prostate cancer, the most widely used system is called the TNM System. It is also known as the Staging System of the American Joint Committee on Cancer (AJCC).

The TNM System describes the extent of the primary tumor (T category), whether the cancer has spread to nearby lymph nodes (N category), and the absence or presence of distant metastasis (M category). The overall stage takes all 3 categories into account, along with the Gleason score (see page 28).

The stages described below are based on the most recent (2002) version of the AJCC staging manual. Some doctors, however, may still be using the 1997 version, which is slightly different. This can be confusing, so be sure to ask which version your doctor is using.

There are actually 2 types of staging for prostate cancer. The **clinical stage** is your doctor's best estimate of the extent of your disease, based on the results of the physical exam (including DRE), lab tests, and any imaging studies you have had. If you have surgery, your doctors can determine the **pathologic stage**, which is based on the surgery and examination of the removed tissue. This means that if you have surgery, the stage of your cancer might actually change afterward (if cancer was found in a place it wasn't suspected, for example).

Both types of staging use the same categories (although the T1 category is not used in pathologic staging).

T categories

There are 4 categories for describing the prostate tumor's (T) stage, ranging from T1 to T4. Most of these have subcategories as well.

T1: Your doctor can't feel the tumor or see it with imaging such as transrectal ultrasound.

- **T1a:** The cancer is found incidentally during a transurethral resection (often abbreviated as TURP) for benign prostatic enlargement. Cancer is present in less than 5% of the tissue removed.
- **T1b:** The cancer is found during a TURP but is present in more than 5% of the tissue removed.
- **T1c:** The cancer is found by needle biopsy that was done because of an elevated PSA.

T2: Your doctor can feel the cancer when a digital rectal exam (DRE) is done, but it still appears to be confined to the prostate gland.

- **T2a:** The cancer is in one half or less of only one side (left or right) of your prostate.
- **T2b:** The cancer is in more than half of only one side (left or right) of your prostate.
- **T2c:** The cancer is in both sides of your prostate.

T3: The cancer has begun to spread outside your prostate and may involve the seminal vesicles.

- **T3a:** The cancer extends outside the prostate but not to the seminal vesicles.
- **T3b:** The cancer has spread to the seminal vesicles.

T4: The cancer has spread to tissues next to your prostate (other than the seminal vesicles), such as the bladder sphincter (muscle that helps control urination), the rectum, and/or the wall of the pelvis.

N categories
There are 2 N categories.

N0: The cancer has not spread to any lymph nodes.

N1: The cancer has spread to one or more regional (nearby) lymph nodes in the pelvis.

M categories
There are 2 main M categories.

M0: The cancer has not spread beyond the regional lymph nodes.

M1: The cancer has spread beyond the regional nodes.

- **M1a:** The cancer has spread to distant (outside of the pelvis) lymph nodes.
- **M1b:** The cancer has spread to the bones.
- **M1c:** The cancer has spread to other organs such as lungs, liver, or brain (with or without bone disease).

Stage Groupings
Once the T, N, and M categories have been determined, this information is combined, along with the Gleason score, in a process called stage grouping. The overall stage is expressed in Roman numerals from I (the least advanced) to IV (the most advanced). This is done to help determine treatment options and the outlook for survival or cure.

Stage I
- T1a, N0, M0, low Gleason score (2 to 4)

Stage II
- T1a, N0, M0, intermediate or high Gleason score (5 to 10)
- T1b, N0, M0, any Gleason score (2 to 10)
- T1c, N0, M0, any Gleason score (2 to 10)
- T2, N0, M0, any Gleason score (2 to 10)

Stage III
- T3, N0, M0, any Gleason score (2 to 10)

Stage IV
- T4, N0, M0, any Gleason score (2 to 10)
- Any T, N1, M0, any Gleason score (2 to 10)
- Any T, any N, M1, any Gleason score (2 to 10)

These stages can be described as follows:

Stage I: The cancer is still within the prostate and has not spread to lymph nodes or elsewhere in the body. The cancer was found during a transurethral resection, it had a low Gleason score (2 to 4), and less than 5% of the tissue was cancerous.

Stage II: The cancer is still within the prostate and has not spread to the lymph nodes or elsewhere in the body, and one of the following applies:

- It was found during a transurethral resection and has an intermediate or high Gleason score (5 or higher), or more than 5% of the tissue contained cancer; or

- It was discovered because of a high PSA level, cannot be felt on digital rectal exam or seen on transrectal ultrasound, and was diagnosed by needle biopsy; or
- It can be felt on digital rectal exam or seen on transrectal ultrasound.

Stage III: The cancer has begun to spread outside the prostate and may have spread to the seminal vesicles, but it has not spread to the lymph nodes or elsewhere in the body.

Stage IV: One or more of the following apply:

- The cancer has spread to tissues next to the prostate (other than the seminal vesicles), such as the bladder's external sphincter (muscle that helps control urination), rectum, and/or the wall of the pelvis; and/or
- It has spread to the lymph nodes; and/or
- It has spread to other, more distant sites in the body.

In addition to the TNM system, other systems have been used to stage prostate cancer. The Whitmore-Jewett system, which stages prostate cancer as A, B, C, or D, was commonly used in the past, but most prostate specialists now use the TNM system. If your doctors use this system, ask them to translate it into the TNM system or to explain how their staging will determine your treatment options.

Treatments and Alternatives

How Is Prostate Cancer Treated?

This information represents the views of the doctors and nurses serving on the American Cancer Society's Cancer Information Database Editorial Board. These views are based on their interpretation of studies published in medical journals, as well as their own professional experience.

This treatment information is not official policy of the Society and is not intended as medical advice to replace the expertise and judgment of your cancer care team. It is intended to help you and your family make informed decisions, together with your doctor.

Your doctor may have reasons for suggesting a treatment plan different from these general treatment options. Don't hesitate to ask him or her questions about your treatment options.

General Comments About Treatment Information

Once your prostate cancer has been diagnosed, graded, and staged, you have a lot to think about before you and your doctor choose a treatment plan. You may feel that you must make a decision quickly, but it is important to give yourself time to absorb the information you have just learned. Ask questions of your cancer care team. Read the section, "What Should You Ask Your Doctor About Prostate Cancer?" (See page 89.)

The treatment you choose for prostate cancer should take into account:

- your age and expected life span
- your feelings about the side effects associated with each treatment
- any other serious health conditions you may have
- the stage and grade of your cancer
- the likelihood that each type of treatment will be curative

You may want to get a second opinion about the best treatment option for your situation, especially if there are several choices available to you. You will want to weigh the benefits of each treatment against its possible outcomes, side effects, and risks.

Expectant Management (Watchful Waiting)

Because prostate cancer often grows very slowly, some men (especially those who are older or have other serious health problems) may never need treatment for their prostate cancer. Instead, their doctors may recommend an approach known as expectant management, or **watchful waiting**.

Watchful waiting involves the close monitoring of the cancer with PSA testing without active treatment such as surgery or radiation therapy. It may be recommended if your cancer is not causing any symptoms, is expected to grow very slowly, and is small and contained within one area of the prostate. One recommendation is to measure how quickly the PSA level doubles. If it doubles in less than 3 years, some doctors would recommend treatment.

Watchful waiting is less likely to be an option if you are younger, healthy, and have a fast-growing cancer (for example, a high Gleason score). In a large group of men who were watched without treatment, most did not experience problems with their cancer till after 10 to 15 years.

At this time, watchful waiting is a reasonable option for some men with slow-growing cancers because it is not known if active treatment in these men, such as surgery, radiation therapy, and hormone therapy (described below), prolongs survival. Also, active treatment carries definite risks and side effects that may sometimes outweigh the possible benefits. Some men choose watchful waiting for this reason. Others are not comfortable with this approach, and are willing to accept the possible side effects of active treatments in order to try to remove or destroy the cancer.

Expectant therapy does not mean that you will not receive medical care or follow-up. Rather, your cancer will be carefully observed and monitored. Usually this approach includes a PSA blood test and digital rectal examination (DRE) every 6 months, possibly with yearly transrectal ultrasound-guided biopsy of the prostate. If you develop bothersome symptoms or your cancer begins to grow more quickly, you can consider active treatment.

Hopefully we will have a better idea of the pros and cons of watchful waiting versus active treatment in the near future. A large study sponsored by the US National Cancer Institute and the Veterans Affairs Cooperative

Studies Program is now looking into how active treatment affects survival and quality of life of prostate cancer patients of different ages. The PIVOT (short for Prostatic Intervention Versus Observation Trial) is still in progress.

Surgery

Radical prostatectomy is surgery that attempts to cure prostate cancer. It is used most often if the cancer is not thought to have spread outside of the gland (stage T1 or T2 cancers). In this operation, your surgeon is trying to cure you by removing the entire prostate gland plus some surrounding tissue (including the seminal vesicles).

Radical retropubic prostatectomy

This is the operation used by most urologic surgeons (urologists). You will be either under general anesthesia (asleep) or be given spinal or epidural anesthesia (the same type of anesthesia often given to women during childbirth to numb the lower half of the body) along with sedation during the surgery.

For this operation, the surgeon makes a skin incision in your lower abdomen, from the belly button down to the pubic bone. Some surgeons remove lymph nodes from around the prostate at this time. If any of the nodes contain cancer cells, which means the cancer has spread, they often will not continue with the surgery because it is unlikely that the cancer can be cured.

Other surgeons only remove the prostate gland and may not remove lymph nodes. The decision depends on your PSA level and Gleason score. If either is high, they might remove the lymph nodes around the prostate.

The surgeon will also pay close attention to the 2 tiny bundles of nerves that run on either side of the prostate. These nerves control erections. If they are both removed, you will be impotent (unable to have a spontaneous erection and will require additional treatments to achieve erections). If neither is removed, then you may be able to function normally. Usually this takes a few months after surgery because the nerves have been handled during the operation and won't work properly for a while. If one is removed, you still have a chance of keeping your ability to have an erection, but it is lower than if neither was removed. If you were able to have erections before the surgery, the surgeon will try not to injure these nerves. Of course if the cancer is growing into them, then the surgeon will remove them.

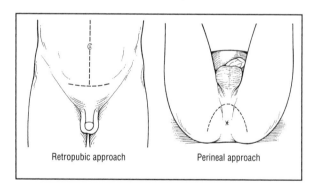

Retropubic approach   Perineal approach

Radical perineal prostatectomy

In this operation, the surgeon makes the incision in the perineum, the skin between the anus and scrotum. This procedure is used less often because the nerves cannot easily be spared and lymph nodes can't be removed. But it is often a shorter operation and might be appropriate if you don't want the nerve-sparing procedure or require lymph node removal. It also might be used if you have other medical conditions that make retropubic surgery difficult for you. It can be just as curative as the retropubic operation if performed correctly.

These operations usually last from $1\frac{1}{2}$ to 4 hours. The perineal operation usually takes less time than the retropubic operation, and may result in less pain afterward. After surgery you will stay in the hospital about 3 days and will probably be away from work for about 3 to 5 weeks.

In most cases, you will be able to donate your own blood before surgery. If needed, this blood can be given back to you during the operation.

After the surgery, while you are still under anesthesia, a catheter will be put in your penis to help drain your bladder. The catheter usually stays in place for 1 to 3 weeks and allows you to urinate easily while you are healing. You will be able to urinate on your own after the catheter is removed.

Laparoscopic radical prostatectomy

Both of the surgical approaches above use an "open" technique, in which the surgeon makes a long incision to remove the prostate. A newer technique, known as **laparoscopic radical prostatectomy** (LRP), involves using several smaller incisions and specialized long instruments to remove the prostate. It is being increasingly used in the United States.

Laparoscopic prostatectomy has advantages over the historical open radical prostatectomy, including less blood loss and pain, and shorter hospital stays (usually no more than a day) and recovery times. LRP is a technically complex operation. In experienced hands, LRP is as efficient as open radical prostatectomy although it takes a bit longer to do. Because LRP offers very good illumination and magnification, LRP is associated with greater precision and control than open radical prostatectomy.

A nerve-sparing approach is possible with LRP, increasing the chance of potency after the operation.

Early studies report that the rates of side effects from LRP seem to be about the same as for open prostatectomy.

Some surgeons do LRP remotely and indirectly by use of a robotic interface (the da Vinci system). For the patient, there is no difference between direct and remote LRP. The choice of direct or remote/indirect LRP reflects surgeon's preference of tools, much as use of needle or sewing machine might reflect the preferences of a seamstress. Far more than choice of instruments, the factor most determining clinical success is the surgeon's experience, commitment, and focus.

LRP has been used in the United States since 1999 and is done in community and university centers. Because it is still relatively new, results of long-term studies are not available. However, one should realize that LRP is not really a new treatment, but rather a modern incarnation of the oldest treatment for prostate cancer: radical prostatectomy.

If you are considering treatment with LRP, it's important to understand what is known and what is not yet known about this approach. If you decide that LRP is the treatment for you, be sure to find a surgeon with a lot of experience doing LRP.

Transurethral resection of the prostate (TURP)

This operation is palliative, which means it is done to relieve symptoms, not to cure. This surgery may be used if you are having trouble urinating because of the cancer and are not a candidate for curative surgery. TURP is also (more commonly) used to treat men with non-cancerous enlargement of the prostate called benign prostatic hyperplasia (BPH).

During this operation, the surgeon removes part of the prostate gland that surrounds the urethra (the tube through which urine exits the bladder). The skin is not cut with this surgery. An instrument called a resecto-scope is passed through the end of the penis into the urethra at the level of the prostate. Once it is in place, electricity is passed through a wire to heat it and cut or vaporize the tissue. Either spinal anesthesia or general anesthesia is used.

The operation usually takes about 1 hour. After surgery, a catheter is inserted through the penis into the bladder. It remains in place for 1 to 3 days to help urine drain while the prostate heals. You can usually leave the hospital after 1 to 2 days and return to work in 1 to 2 weeks. You will likely have some bleeding in the urine after surgery. Other risks include infection and the risks associated with the type of anesthesia used.

Surgical Risks and Possible Side Effects of Radical Prostatectomy

Surgical risks

The risks associated with radical prostatectomy are similar to those of any major surgery, including risks from anesthesia. Among the most serious, there is a small risk of heart attack, stroke, blood clots in the legs that may travel to your lungs, and infection at the incision site. Because there are many blood vessels near the prostate gland, another risk is bleeding during and after the surgery. You may need blood product transfusions, which carry their own small risk. In extremely rare cases, people die because of complications of this operation. Your risk depends, in part, on your overall health, your age, and the skill of your surgical team.

The major possible **side effects** of radical prostatectomy are urinary incontinence and impotence. It should be noted that these side effects are also possible with other forms of therapy, although they are described here in more detail. One minor effect may be a decrease in penis length. In one study, about 20% of men had a 15% decrease in the length of their penis.

Urinary incontinence

You might develop urinary **incontinence**, which means you can't control your urine or have leakage or dribbling. There are different degrees of incontinence. Being incontinent can affect you not only physically but emotionally and socially as well.

There are 3 types of incontinence:

- Men with **stress incontinence** leak urine when they cough, laugh, sneeze, or exercise. It is usually caused by problems with the bladder sphincter (the muscular valve that keeps urine in the bladder). Prostate cancer treatments may damage the muscles that form this valve or the nerves that keep the muscle working. Stress incontinence is the most common type of incontinence after prostate surgery.

- Men with **overflow incontinence** take a long time to urinate and have a dribbling stream with little force. Overflow incontinence is usually caused by blockage or narrowing of the bladder outlet by cancer or scar tissue.
- Men with **urge incontinence** have a sudden need to go to the bathroom and pass urine. This problem occurs when the bladder becomes too sensitive to stretching by urine accumulation.

For many patients with prostate cancer, normal bladder control returns within several weeks or months after radical prostatectomy. This recovery usually occurs gradually, in stages.

Unfortunately, doctors can't predict how any man will function after surgery. In one large study of men treated in all different types of hospitals, researchers found that 5 years after radical prostatectomy:

- 14% of the men had no bladder control or had frequent leaks or dripping of urine
- 16% leaked more than twice a day
- 29% wore pads to keep dry

Most large cancer centers, where prostate surgery is done more often and surgeons have more experience in performing radical prostatectomies, report fewer problems with incontinence.

Treatment of incontinence depends on its type, cause, and severity. If you have problems with incontinence, let your doctors know. You might feel embarrassed about discussing this issue, but remember that you are not alone. This is a common medical problem. Doctors who treat men with prostate cancer should be very knowledgeable about incontinence and should be able to suggest ways to improve this condition.

Your doctor may recommend special exercises, called **Kegel exercises**, to help strengthen your bladder muscles. These exercises involve tensing and relaxing certain pelvic muscles. Not all doctors agree as to their usefulness or as to the best way to do them, so ask your doctor about doing Kegels before you try them.

There are also *medicines* to help the muscles of the bladder or sphincter. Most of these medicines affect either the muscles or the nerves that control them. These are more effective for some forms of incontinence than for others.

Surgery may also be used to correct long-term incontinence. Material such as collagen can be injected by surgery to tighten the bladder sphincter. If your incontinence is severe and persistent, an artificial sphincter can be implanted surgically, or a small device called a urethral sling may be implanted to keep the bladder neck where it belongs. Ask your doctor if these treatments might help you.

If your incontinence cannot be completely corrected, it can still be helped. You can learn how to manage and live with your incontinence. Incontinence is more than a physical problem. It can disrupt your quality of life if it is not managed well.

There is no one right way to cope with incontinence. The challenge is to find what works for you so that you can return to your normal daily activities. There are many *incontinence products* to help keep you mobile and comfortable such as pads that are worn under your clothing. Adult briefs and adult undergarments are bulkier than pads but provide more protection. Bed pads or absorbent mattress covers can also be used to protect the bed linens and mattress.

When choosing incontinence products, keep in mind the checklist below. Some of these questions may not be important to you, or you may have others to add.

- *Absorbency:* How much does the product provide? How long will it protect?
- *Bulk:* Can it be seen under normal clothing? Is it disposable? Or reusable?
- *Comfort:* How does it feel when you move or sit down?
- *Availability:* Which stores carry the product? Are they easy to get to?
- *Cost:* Does your insurance pay for these products?

There are also sheaths called condom catheters as well as compression devices that are placed on the penis for short periods of time. For some types of incontinence, self-catheterization may be an option. In this approach, you insert a thin tube into your urethra to drain and empty the bladder. It is easy to learn this safe and usually painless technique. Talk with your doctor about the best methods for dealing with your incontinence.

Also, you can follow some simple precautions that make incontinence less of a problem. For example, empty your bladder before bedtime or before strenuous or vigorous activity. Avoid drinking too much fluid, particularly if the drinks contain caffeine or alcohol, which can make you have to go more often. Because fat in the abdomen can push on the bladder, losing weight sometimes helps improve bladder control.

Fear, anxiety, and anger are common feelings for people dealing with incontinence. Fear of having an accident may keep you from doing the things you enjoy most—taking your grandchild to the park, going to the movies, or playing a round of golf. You may feel isolated and embarrassed. You may even avoid sex because you are afraid of leakage. Be sure and talk to your doctor so you can begin to solve the problem.

Impotence

Impotence, also known as **erectile dysfunction**, means you cannot get an erection sufficient for sexual penetration. The nerves that allow men to get erections may be damaged or removed by radical prostatectomy. Radiation therapy and cryosurgery can also damage these nerves.

During the first 3 to 12 months after radical prostatectomy, you will probably not be able to have a spontaneous erection, so you may need to use medicines or other treatments. Your ability to achieve an erection after surgery will be related to your age, your ability to get an erection before the operation, and whether the nerves were cut. You should expect some decrease in your ability to have an erection, but the younger you are, the more likely it is that you will retain more of this ability.

Some cancer centers that perform many radical nerve-sparing prostatectomies report that the impotence rate is as low as 25% to 30% for men under 60. However, other doctors have reported higher rates of impotence in similar patients. Impotence occurs in 70% to 80% of men over 70, even if nerves on both sides are not removed. If potency remains after surgery, the sensation of orgasm should continue to be pleasurable, but there is no ejaculation of semen. The orgasm is "dry." In the study quoted above, three fourths of men were unable to have erections satisfactory for intercourse after radical prostatectomy. But these numbers do not distinguish between those who were impotent before treatment and those who weren't. When the study looked at men with normal sexual function before surgery, they found that nearly half had lost sexual function.

Most doctors feel that regaining potency is helped along by attempting to get an erection as soon as possible once the body has had a chance to heal (usually about 6 weeks after the operation). Medication (see below) may be helpful at this time. Be sure to talk to your doctor for recommendations in your particular situation.

Several options may help you if you have erectile dysfunction.

Phosphodiesterase inhibitors, such as sildenafil (Viagra), vardenafil (Levitra), and tadalafil (Cialis) are pills that can promote erections. These drugs will not work if both nerves have been damaged or removed. The most common side effects are headache, flushing (skin becoming red and feeling warm), indigestion, light sensitivity and other visual problems, and runny or stuffy nose. Nitrates, drugs used often as treatment for heart disease, can interact with these drugs to cause very low blood pressure, a complication that can be fatal, so be sure your doctor knows which medicines you are taking.

Another problem with these drugs is loss of vision. Some medical journal articles have indicated that Viagra and other medications for treating erectile dysfunction in men could in very rare cases cause blockage of blood flow to the optic nerve in the inner back of the eye, which could lead to blindness. Men who developed this complication often had pre-existing high blood pressure, diabetes, elevated cholesterol, or high levels of fat in their blood (hyperlipidemia).

Prostaglandin E1 is a substance naturally made in the body that can produce erections. It can be injected almost painlessly into the base of the penis 5 to 10 minutes before intercourse or introduced into the urethra as a suppository. You can even increase the dosage to prolong the erection. You may experience side effects, such as pain, dizziness, and prolonged erection, but they are usually minimal.

Vacuum devices are another option that may create an erection. These mechanical pumps are placed around the entire penis before intercourse to produce an erection.

If other methods do not help, **penile implants** might restore your ability to have erections. There are several types of penile implants, including those using silicone rods or inflatable devices.

Sterility

Aside from the possibility of impotence, radical prostatectomy severs the connection between the testicles (where sperm are produced) and the urethra. This means that a man can no longer father a child. Often, this is not an issue, as men with prostate cancer tend to be older. But if it is a concern for you, you may want to speak with your doctor about "banking" your sperm before the operation.

Lymphedema

A rare but possible complication of removing many of the lymph nodes around the prostate (either surgically or laparoscopically) is a condition called lymphedema. Lymph nodes normally provide a way for fluid to return from all areas of the body to the heart. When nodes are removed, fluid may collect in the legs or genital region over time, leading to swelling and pain. Lymphedema can usually be treated with physical therapy, although it may not disappear completely.

Radiation Therapy

Radiation therapy uses high-energy rays or particles to kill cancer cells. Radiation is sometimes used to treat low-grade cancer that is still confined within the prostate gland or that has only spread to nearby tissue. Cure rates for men with these types of cancers appear to be similar to those for men getting radical prostatectomy. If the disease is more advanced, radiation may be used to reduce the size of the tumor and to provide relief from present and possible future symptoms.

Two main types of radiation therapy are used: external beam radiation and brachytherapy (internal radiation). Both appear to be good methods of treating prostate cancer, although there is more long-term information about the results of treatment with external beam radiation.

External Beam Radiation Therapy (EBRT)

In this technique, radiation is focused on the prostate gland from a source outside your body. It is much like getting a diagnostic x-ray but for a longer time. Before treatments start, imaging studies such as

MRIs, CT scans, or plain x-rays of the pelvis are done to find the exact location of your prostate gland. The radiation team will then make some ink marks on your skin that they will use later as a guide to focus the radiation in the right area. You will usually be treated 5 days per week in an outpatient center over a period of 8 or 9 weeks. Each treatment lasts only a few minutes and is painless.

Aside from being used as an initial treatment for early stage cancer, external beam radiation can also be used to help relieve bone pain when the cancer has spread to a specific area of bone.

Newer forms of external beam radiation appear promising for increasing the success rate and reducing side effects.

Three-dimensional conformal radiation therapy (3DCRT) uses special computers to precisely map the location of your prostate. You are fitted with a plastic mold resembling a body cast to keep you still so that the radiation can be aimed more accurately. Radiation beams are then aimed at the prostate from several directions, which makes it less likely to damage normal tissues.

Although the procedure is relatively new, the short-term results suggest that it is at least as effective as standard radiation therapy, so many doctors now recommend using it when it is available. In theory, by aiming the radiation more accurately, doctors can reduce radiation damage to tissues near the prostate and cure more cancers by increasing the radiation dose to the prostate. Long-term study results are needed to confirm this, however.

Intensity modulated radiation therapy (IMRT) is an advanced form of 3D therapy. It uses a machine that actually moves around the patient as it delivers radiation. In addition to aiming beams from several directions, the intensity (or strength) of the beams can be adjusted to minimize the dose of radiation reaching the most sensitive normal tissues while delivering a uniformly high dose to the cancer. Many major hospitals and cancer centers are able to provide IMRT.

Conformal proton beam radiation therapy, a technique related to 3DCRT, uses a similar approach. But instead of using x-rays, this technique focuses proton beams on the cancer. **Protons** are positive parts of atoms that cause little damage to tissues they pass through but are effective in killing cells at the end of their path. This means that proton beam radiation may be able to deliver more radiation to the prostate while reducing side effects on nearby normal tissues. As with 3DCRT, preliminary results are promising, but a long-term advantage over standard external beam radiation has not yet been proven. Also, proton beam radiation may not be covered by all insurance companies, and there are only 3 proton beam devices in the United States (California, Indiana, Massachusetts) at this time, with 2 more planned to open in 2006 (Texas, Florida).

Possible Side Effects of External Beam Radiation Therapy

The numbers used in describing the possible side effects below relate to conventional external radiation therapy. The risks of the newer techniques described above are likely to be lower.

Bowel problems: During treatment with external beam radiation therapy, you may develop diarrhea, sometimes with blood in the stool, rectal leakage, and an irritated large intestine. Occasionally, normal bowel function does not return after treatment ends. In one study, about 10% to 20% of men reported these types of bowel problems, such as pain, burning, and/or diarrhea, after their external beam radiation therapy. The newer technique of conformal radiation therapy may lessen these complications.

Bladder problems: You might also have trouble with frequent urination, a burning sensation while urinating, and blood in your urine. Bladder problems persist in about one-third of patients, with the most common problem being frequent urination. About 2% to 5% of men treated with external beam radiation therapy reported long-term use of absorbent pads for incontinence.

Incontinence: Although this side effect is less common than after surgery, a recent study found that the number of incontinent men continued to increase every year after radiation; by 6 years after treatment, the rate was almost as high as it was in men who had surgery.

Impotence: After several years, the impotence rate after radiation is the same as that of surgery. It usually does not occur right after radiation therapy but gradually develops over a year or more. About 77% of men are impotent within 5 years of having external beam radiation therapy. In men who had normal potency before treatment, about half become impotent at 5 years. This is different from surgery, where impotence occurs immediately and may improve over time. As with surgery, the older you are, the more likely it is you will become impotent. The impotence may be helped by treatments such as phosphodiesterase inhibitors (see the surgery section for more details). A recent study of men who were impotent after radiation treatment for prostate cancer found that over half had erections after using sildenafil (Viagra).

Radiation therapy may also cause fatigue that may not disappear until a few months after treatment stops. **Lymphedema** is another possibility.

Brachytherapy (Internal Radiation Therapy)

Brachytherapy (also called seed implantation or interstitial radiation therapy) uses small radioactive pellets, or "seeds," each about the size of a grain of rice, that are placed directly into your prostate. Brachytherapy is generally used only in men with early stage prostate cancer that is relatively slow growing.

Its use may also be limited by other factors. For men who have undergone a transurethral resection of the prostate (TURP) or those who already have urinary problems, the risk of urinary side effects may be higher. The same is true for men with large prostate glands. Doctors are now studying ways of getting around this, such as giving men a short course of hormone therapy beforehand to shrink the prostate.

Imaging tests such as transrectal ultrasound, CT scans, or MRI help guide the placement of the radio-active pellets. Special computer programs calculate the exact dose of radiation needed. Without these, your cancer might receive too little radiation or the sur-rounding benign tissues could receive too much.

There are 2 types of prostate brachytherapy. Both are done in an operating room and require some type of anesthesia.

For *permanent (low dose rate, or LDR) brachytherapy,* pellets of radioactive material (isotopes such as iodine-125 or palladium-103) are placed inside thin needles, which are inserted through the skin of the perineum (area between the scrotum and anus) into the prostate. The pellets (seeds) are left in place as the needles are removed and give off low doses of radiation for weeks or months.

Usually, anywhere from 40 to 100 seeds are placed. Because they are so small, their presence causes little discomfort, and they are simply left in place after their radioactive material is used up. This type of radiation therapy requires spinal or general anesthesia and may require 1 day in the hospital.

You may also receive external beam radiation with brachytherapy, especially if there is a risk that your cancer has spread outside of the prostate (for example, if you have a high Gleason score).

Temporary (high dose rate, or HDR) brachytherapy is a newer technique. Hollow needles are placed through the perineum into the prostate. Radioactive iridium-192 is then placed in the needles, usually for 5 to 15 minutes. Generally, about 3 brief treatments are given, and the iridium is removed each time. The treatments are usually given over a couple of days. For about a week following insertion of the needles, you may have some pain in the area between your scrotum and rectum, and your urine may be reddish-brown. Recently, cesium 137 has become available as another isotope to use in brachytherapy.

These treatments are usually combined with external beam radiation given at a lower dose than it normally would be if used by itself. The total dose of radiation is high enough to kill all the cancer cells. The advantage is that most of the radiation is concentrated in the prostate gland itself, sparing the urethra and the tissues around the prostate such as the nerves, bladder, and rectum.

Possible Risks and Side Effects of Brachytherapy

If you receive permanent brachytherapy seeds, they will give off small amounts of radiation for several weeks. Even though the radiation doesn't travel far, you may be told to stay away from pregnant women and small children during this time. You may be asked to take other precautions as well, such as wearing a condom during sex.

There is also a small risk that some of the seeds may move (migrate). You may be asked to strain your urine for the first week or so to catch any seeds that might come out. Be sure to carefully follow any instructions your doctor gives you. There have also been reports of the seeds migrating to other parts of the body such as the lungs, although as far as doctors can tell, these don't seem to cause any ill effects.

Like external beam radiation, brachytherapy can also cause impotence, urinary problems, and bowel problems. Significant long-term bowel problems (including burning and rectal pain and/or diarrhea) occur in less than 5% of patients.

Severe urinary incontinence is not a common side effect. But **frequent urination** may persist in about one-third of patients who have brachytherapy. This is perhaps caused by irritation of the urethra, the tube that drains urine from the bladder. This may actually close off (known as urethral stricture) and need to be opened with surgery.

Impotence may be less likely to develop after brachytherapy, but it is unclear. Brachytherapy wasn't evaluated in the study mentioned above, but another major study (CaPSURE) rates brachytherapy as having the lowest rate of sexual dysfunction, even after 5 years. But another study that followed men for over 6 years found that their impotence rate was no lower than with external beam radiation or surgery.

Cryosurgery

Cryosurgery (also called cryotherapy or cryoablation) is sometimes used to treat localized prostate cancer by freezing the prostate. As with brachytherapy, this may not be a good option for men with large prostate glands.

Several hollow probes (needles) are placed through the skin between the anus and scrotum. The doctor guides them into the prostate using transrectal ultrasound (TRUS). Very cold gases are passed through the needles, creating ice balls that destroy the prostate gland. To be sure prostate tissue is destroyed without too much damage to nearby tissues, the doctor carefully watches the ultrasound images during the procedure. Warm saltwater is circulated through a catheter in the urethra to keep it from freezing. Spinal, epidural, or general anesthesia is used during the procedure.

A suprapubic catheter is placed through a skin incision on the abdomen into the bladder so that if the prostate swells after the procedure (which usually occurs), it won't block the passage of urine. The catheter is removed a couple of weeks later, once urination returns to normal. After the procedure, there will be some bruising and soreness of the area where the probe was inserted. You will likely stay in the hospital for a day.

Cryosurgery is less invasive than radical prostatectomy, so there is less blood loss, a shorter hospital stay, shorter recovery period, and less pain than with surgery. But compared with surgery or radiation therapy, doctors know much less about the long-term effectiveness of cryosurgery. Current techniques using ultrasound guidance and precise temperature monitoring have only been available for a few years. Outcomes of long-term (10- to 15-year) follow-up must still be collected and analyzed. For this reason, most doctors do not include cryotherapy among the options they routinely consider for initial treatment of prostate cancer. It is sometimes recommended if the cancer has come back after other treatment.

Possible Side Effects of Cryosurgery

Side effects from cryosurgery tend to be worse if the procedure is being done in men who have already received radiation therapy, as opposed to men who receive it as the first form of treatment.

Most men have blood in their urine for a day or two after the procedure, as well as soreness in the area where the needles were placed. Swelling of the penis or scrotum is also common. The freezing may also affect the bladder and intestines, which can lead to pain, burning sensations, and the need to empty the bladder and bowels often. Most men recover normal bowel and bladder function over time.

Freezing damages nerves near the prostate and causes **impotence** in most men who have cryosurgery. This complication probably occurs more often after cryosurgery than it does after radical prostatectomy (see page 48).

Urinary incontinence is rare in men for whom cryosurgery is the primary treatment for prostate cancer, but it is more common in men who have already had radiation therapy.

A fistula (abnormal opening or connection) between the rectum and bladder develops in about 2% of men after cryosurgery. This can allow urine to leak into the rectum, and may require surgery to repair.

Hormone (Androgen Deprivation) Therapy

The goal of **hormone therapy** (also called **androgen deprivation therapy** [ADT] or androgen suppression therapy) is to lower levels of the male hormones (androgens, mainly testosterone) in the body. Androgens, produced mainly in the testicles, stimulate prostate cancer cells to grow. Lowering androgen levels often makes prostate cancers shrink or grow more slowly. But hormone therapy does not cure prostate cancer and is not a substitute for curative treatment.

Hormone therapy may be used in several situations:

- as first-line (initial) therapy if you are not able to have surgery or radiation or can't be cured by these treatments because the cancer has already spread beyond the prostate gland
- after initial treatment, such as surgery or radiation therapy, if the cancer remains or comes back

- as an addition (adjuvant) to radiation therapy as initial treatment in certain groups of men at high risk for cancer recurrence
- before surgery or radiation (neoadjuvant therapy), in an attempt to shrink the cancer and make the other treatment more effective

Types of Hormone Therapy

There are several methods used for androgen suppression therapy.

Orchiectomy: In this operation, the surgeon removes the testicles, where more than 90% of the androgens, mostly testosterone, are produced. With this source removed, most prostate cancers shrink. It is done as a simple outpatient procedure. This is probably the least expensive and simplest way to reduce androgen production. However, unlike some of the other methods of lowering androgen levels, it is permanent, and many men have trouble accepting the removal of their testicles. For those men having the procedure, silicone prostheses that resemble testes can be inserted into the scrotal sac if they wish.

Possible **side effects** of orchiectomy are generally related to changing levels of hormones in the body. About 90% of men who have had this operation have reduced or absent libido (sexual desire) and impotence. Some men also experience:

- hot flashes (these may go away with time)
- breast tenderness and growth of breast tissue
- osteoporosis (weakening of bones) leading to bone fractures
- anemia (low red blood cell counts)
- decreased mental acuity

- loss of muscle mass
- weight gain
- fatigue
- decrease in HDL ("good") cholesterol
- depression

Many of these side effects can be treated. Sometimes the hot flashes will be improved by treatment with the antidepressants called SSRI inhibitors. Prozac is an example. Brief radiation treatment to the breasts can prevent their enlargement. The osteoporosis can be a major problem because these men are more likely to develop bone fractures. They should be carefully observed and if osteoporosis develops, they should be treated. There are several different drugs available. Exercise is a good way to reduce the chance of loss of muscle mass, fatigue, and decrease weight gain. Usually, the anemia is very mild and doesn't cause symptoms. Depression can be treated by antidepressants.

Luteinizing hormone-releasing hormone (LHRH) analogs: Even though **LHRH analogs** (also called **LHRH agonists**) are more expensive and require more frequent doctor visits, most men choose this method over orchiectomy. These drugs lower testosterone levels as effectively as orchiectomy by decreasing the androgens, mainly testosterone, produced by your testicles.

LHRH analogs are injected or placed as small implants under the skin. They are given either monthly or every 3, 4, 6, or 12 months. The LHRH analogs currently available in the United States include leuprolide (Lupron, Viadur, Eligard), goserelin (Zoladex), and triptorelin (Trelstar).

Possible **side effects** of LHRH analogs such as hot flashes, osteoporosis, and others are similar to those of orchiectomy, and are largely due to low testosterone levels.

When LHRH analogs are first given, testosterone production increases briefly before decreasing to very low levels. This effect is called **flare** and results from the complex way in which LHRH analogs work. Men whose cancer has spread to the bones may experience bone pain. If the cancer has spread to the spine, even a temporary increase in growth could compress the spinal cord and cause pain or paralysis. Flare can be avoided by giving antiandrogens for a few weeks when starting treatment with LHRH analogs.

Luteinizing hormone-releasing hormone (LHRH) antagonists: A newer drug, abarelix (Plenaxis), is an LHRH antagonist. It is thought to work in a way similar to LHRH agonists, but it appears to lower testosterone levels more quickly and does not cause tumor flare like the LHRH agonists do.

However, in clinical trials, a small percentage of men (less than 5%) had serious allergic reactions to the drug. Because of this, it is only approved for use in men who have serious symptoms from advanced prostate cancer and who cannot or refuse to take other forms of hormone therapy.

The possible side effects are similar to those with orchiectomy (see above) or LHRH agonists.

Abarelix is given only in qualified doctors' offices. It is injected into the buttocks every 2 weeks for the first month, then every 4 weeks. You will be asked to remain in the office for 30 minutes after the injection to make sure you are not having an allergic reaction.

Antiandrogens: Antiandrogens block the body's ability to use any androgens. Even after orchiectomy or during treatment with LHRH analogs, a small amount of androgens is still produced by the adrenal glands.

Drugs of this type, such as flutamide (Eulexin), bicalutamide (Casodex), and nilutamide (Nilandron), are taken daily as pills.

Antiandrogen treatment is often combined with orchiectomy or LHRH analogs. This combination is called **combined androgen blockade** (CAB). There is still some debate as to whether CAB is more effective than using orchiectomy or an LHRH analog alone. If there is a benefit, it appears to be small.

An antiandrogen may be added if treatment with orchiectomy or an LHRH analog is no longer working by itself.

Some doctors are testing the use of antiandrogens instead of orchiectomy or LHRH analogs. Several recent studies have compared the effectiveness of antiandrogens alone with that of LHRH agonists. Most found no difference in survival rates, but a few found antiandrogens to be slightly less effective.

If hormone therapy including an antiandrogen becomes ineffective, some men seem to benefit for a short time from simply stopping the antiandrogen. Doctors call this the "antiandrogen withdrawal" effect, although they are not sure why it happens.

Side effects of antiandrogens in patients already treated by orchiectomy or with LHRH agonists are usually not serious. Diarrhea is the major side effect, although nausea, liver problems, and tiredness can also occur. The major difference from LHRH agonists is that antiandrogens have fewer sexual side effects. Libido and potency can be maintained on these drugs if they are used alone.

Other androgen-suppressing drugs: Estrogens, such as diethylstilbestrol (DES), were once the main alternative to orchiectomy for men with advanced prostate cancer. Because of their possible side effects (including blood clots and breast enlargement), estrogens have been largely replaced by LHRH analogs and antiandrogens, although estrogens may be tried if androgen deprivation is no longer effective.

Ketoconazole (Nizoral), first used for treating fungal infections, blocks production of androgens and is sometimes used.

Current Controversies in Hormone Therapy

Many issues surrounding hormone therapy are not yet resolved, such as the best time to start and stop it and the best way to give it. Studies addressing these issues are now underway.

Early vs. delayed treatment: Some doctors think that hormone therapy works better if it is started as soon as possible once the cancer has reached an advanced stage (for example, spread to lymph nodes), or is large (T3) or has a high Gleason score, even though the patient feels well. Some studies have shown that several years of androgen deprivation leads to better outcomes in terms of slower progression and perhaps even longer survival. But not all doctors agree. Some feel that because of the possible side effects and the chance that the cancer could become resistant to therapy sooner, treatment should not be started until symptoms from the disease appear.

Intermittent vs. continuous hormone therapy: Nearly all prostate cancers treated with hormone therapy become resistant to this treatment over a period of months or years. Some doctors believe that constant androgen suppression may not be necessary, so they recommend intermittent (on-again, off-again) treatment.

In one form of intermittent therapy, androgen suppression is stopped once your blood PSA level drops to a very low level. If your PSA level begins to rise, the drugs are started again. Another form of intermittent therapy involves using androgen suppression for fixed periods of time—for example, 6 months on followed by 6 months off.

Clinical trials of intermittent hormonal therapy are still in progress, and it is too early to say whether this new approach is better or worse than continuous hormonal therapy. However, one advantage of intermittent treatment is that for a while some men are able to avoid the side effects of hormonal therapy such as impotence, hot flashes, and loss of sex drive.

Combined androgen blockade: Sometimes, patients have been treated with both androgen deprivation, such as and LHRH agonists, along with an antiandrogen. So far, there has been no conclusive evidence that this combined therapy is better than one drug alone.

Chemotherapy

Chemotherapy is sometimes used if prostate cancer has spread outside of the prostate gland and hormone therapy isn't working. It is not recommended as a treatment if you have early prostate cancer.

Chemotherapy uses anticancer drugs injected into a vein or given by mouth. These drugs enter the bloodstream and reach throughout the body, making this treatment potentially useful for cancers that have spread (metastasized) to distant organs.

Until recently, chemotherapy has not been very effective in treating prostate cancer. In the past few years, the chemotherapy drug mitoxantrone combined with prednisone, has been shown to palliate symptoms from prostate cancer in men with advanced disease. A combination of the chemotherapy drug docetaxel (Taxotere) and prednisone have been shown to prolong life (compared with mitoxantrone/prednisone) in patients with advanced prostate cancer who have failed hormone therapy and is considered the best first chemotherapy option in men whose cancer is no longer responding to hormonal treatments.

Some of the other chemotherapy drugs used to treat prostate cancer include:

- doxorubicin
- etoposide
- vinblastine
- paclitaxel
- carboplatin

Like hormone therapy, chemotherapy is unlikely to result in a cure. This treatment is not expected to destroy all the cancer cells, but it may slow the cancer's growth and reduce symptoms, resulting in a better quality of life.

Possible Side Effects of Chemotherapy

Chemotherapy drugs kill cancer cells but also damage some normal cells, which can lead to side effects. The side effects of chemotherapy depend on the type of drugs used, the amount taken, and the length of treatment. Temporary side effects of most chemotherapy drugs might include:

- nausea and vomiting
- loss of appetite
- hair loss
- mouth sores
- increased chance of infection (due to a shortage of white blood cells)
- increased risk of bleeding or bruising (due to a shortage of blood platelets)
- fatigue (due to low red blood cell counts)

In addition, each chemotherapy drug may have its own unique side effects. For example, estramustine, a drug now commonly used to treat prostate cancer, also carries the risk of blood clots.

There are remedies for many of the temporary side effects of chemotherapy. For example, drugs (**antiemetics**) can be given to prevent or reduce nausea and vomiting. Other drugs can be given to boost blood cell counts. Most side effects disappear once treatment stops.

Treatment of Pain and Other Symptoms

Most of this information discusses ways to remove or to destroy prostate cancer cells or to slow their growth. But maintaining your quality of life is another important goal. Don't hesitate to discuss pain, other symptoms, or any quality of life concerns with your cancer care team. Pain and most other symptoms of prostate cancer can often be treated effectively.

When properly prescribed, pain medicines (ranging from aspirin to opioids) are very effective. Although you may worry about addiction or dependence with opioids, these are almost never problems if you have cancer pain. Symptoms such as drowsiness and constipation are possible, but can usually be treated by adjusting doses or by adding other medicines.

Bisphosphonates are a group of drugs that can relieve bone pain caused by cancer that has metastasized. These drugs may also slow the growth of the metastases and prevent fractures. Bisphosphonates may also have the added benefit of strengthening bones in men who are also receiving hormone therapy. Many doctors will give zoledronic acid (Zometa), which is approved for use in bone metastases from prostate cancer. It is given as an intravenous (IV) injection. Other bisphosphonates have been approved for other uses, and some doctors use these "off label" (a drug prescribed to treat a condition for which it has not been approved by the Food and Drug Administration) to treat prostate cancer.

Recently doctors have been reporting damage to the jawbones as a very distressing side effect of patients receiving bisphosphonates. This side effect is called osteonecrosis. Patients complain of pain in the jaw and examining doctors find that part of the bone of the upper or lower jaw has died. This can lead to loss of teeth in that area. Infections of the jaw bone may also develop. Doctors don't know why this happens or how to prevent it. So far, the only treatment has been to stop the bisphosphonate treatment. The only factor that doctors have found that increases the risk of this problem is having jaw surgery or having a tooth removed. These should be avoided.

One way to avoid these dental procedures is to maintain good oral hygiene by flossing, brushing, making sure that dentures fit properly, and having regular dental checkups. Any tooth or gum infections should be treated promptly. Dental fillings, root canal procedures, and tooth crowns do not seem to lead to osteonecrosis. Some oncologists (doctors who specialize in caring for people who have cancer) recommend that patients have a dental checkup and have any tooth or jaw problems treated before they start taking bisphosphonates.

Some studies suggest that corticosteroids (such as prednisone and dexamethasone) can relieve bone pain in some men.

Radiation therapy with external beam radiation and/or radiopharmaceuticals can also be used to relieve bone pain.

Strontium-89 (Metastron) and Samarium-153 (Quadramet) are drugs called **radiopharmaceuticals**. They are not used to treat early stage, localized prostate cancer, but are used to treat bone pain caused by metastatic prostate cancer. Radiopharmaceuticals are a group of drugs that have radioactive elements. They are injected into a vein and attach to bone. Once attached, the radiation they give off kills the cancer cells and relieves some of the pain caused by bone metastases.

About 80% of prostate cancer patients with painful bone metastases are helped by this treatment. If prostate cancer has spread to many bones, this approach is much better than trying to aim external beam radiation at each affected bone. In some cases, they are used together with external beam radiation aimed at the most painful bone metastases.

The major side effect of this treatment is a lowering of blood cell counts, which could place you at increased risk for infections or bleeding, especially if your counts are already low.

It is very important that your pain be treated effectively. This will help you feel better and allow you to concentrate on the things that are important in your life.

Clinical Trials

The purpose of clinical trials

Studies of promising new or experimental treatments in patients are known as **clinical trials**. A clinical trial is only done when there is some reason to believe that the treatment being studied may be valuable to the patient. Treatments used in clinical trials are often found to have real benefits. Researchers conduct studies of new treatments to answer the following questions:

- Is the treatment helpful?
- How does this new type of treatment work?
- Does it work better than other treatments already available?
- What side effects does the treatment cause?
- Are the side effects greater or less than the standard treatment?
- Do the benefits outweigh the side effects?
- In which patients is the treatment most likely to be helpful?

Types of clinical trials

There are 3 phases of clinical trials in which a treatment is studied before it is eligible for approval by the FDA (Food and Drug Administration).

Phase I clinical trials

The purpose of a phase I study is to find the best way to give a new treatment and how much of it can be given safely. The cancer care team watches patients carefully for any harmful side effects. The treatment has been well tested in lab and animal studies, but the side effects in patients are not completely known. Doctors conducting the clinical trial start by giving very low doses of the drug to the first patients and increasing the dose for later groups of patients until side effects appear. Although doctors are hoping to help patients, the main purpose of a phase I study is to test the safety of the drug.

Phase II clinical trials

These studies are designed to see if the drug works. Patients are given the highest dose that doesn't cause severe side effects (determined from the phase I study) and closely observed for an effect on the cancer. The cancer care team also looks for side effects.

Phase III clinical trials

Phase III studies involve large numbers of patients —often several hundred. One group (the control group) receives the standard (most accepted) treatment. The other group receives the new treatment. All patients in phase III studies are closely watched. The study will be stopped if the side effects of the new treatment are too severe or if one group has had much better results than the others.

If you are in a clinical trial, you will have a team of experts taking care of you and monitoring your progress very carefully. The study is especially designed to pay close attention to you.

However, there are some risks. No one involved in the study knows in advance whether the treatment will work or exactly what side effects will occur. That is what the study is designed to find out. While most side effects disappear in time, some can be permanent or even life threatening. Keep in mind, though, that even standard treatments have side effects. Depending on many factors, you may decide to enroll in a clinical trial.

Deciding to enter a clinical trial

Enrollment in any clinical trial is completely up to you. Your doctors and nurses will explain the study to you in detail and will give you a form to read and sign indicating your desire to take part. This process is known as giving your informed consent. Even after signing the form and after the clinical trial begins, you are free to leave the study at any time, for any reason. Taking part in the study does not prevent you from getting other medical care you may need.

To find out more about clinical trials, ask your cancer care team. Among the questions you should ask are:

- Is there a clinical trial for which I would be eligible?
- What is the purpose of the study?
- What kinds of tests and treatments does the study involve?
- What does this treatment do? Has it been used before?
- Will I know which treatment I receive?
- What is likely to happen in my case with, or without, this new treatment?

- What are my other choices and their advantages and disadvantages?
- How could the study affect my daily life?
- What side effects can I expect from the study? Can the side effects be controlled?
- Will I have to be hospitalized? If so, how often and for how long?
- Will the study cost me anything? Will any of the treatment be free?
- If I am harmed as a result of the research, what treatment would I be entitled to?
- What type of long-term follow-up care is part of the study?
- Has the treatment been used to treat other types of cancers?

The American Cancer Society offers a clinical trials matching service for patients, their family, and friends. You can reach this service at 1-800-303-5691 or on our Web site at http://clinicaltrials.cancer.org. Based on the information you provide about your cancer type, stage, and previous treatments, this service can compile a list of clinical trials that match your medical needs. In finding a center most convenient for you, the service can also take into account where you live and whether you are willing to travel.

You can also get a list of current clinical trials by calling the National Cancer Institute's Cancer Information Service toll free at 1-800-4-CANCER or by visiting the NCI clinical trials Web site at www.cancer.gov/clinical_trials/.

Complementary and Alternative Methods

Complementary and alternative therapies are a diverse group of health care practices, systems, and products that are not part of usual medical treatment. They may include products such as vitamins, herbs, or dietary supplements, or procedures such as acupuncture, massage, and a host of other types of treatment. There is a great deal of interest today in complementary and alternative treatments for cancer. Many are now being studied to find out if they are truly helpful to people with cancer.

You may hear about different treatments from family, friends, and others, which may be offered as a way to treat your cancer or to help you feel better. Some of these treatments are harmless in certain situations, while others have been shown to cause harm. Most of them are of unproven benefit.

The American Cancer Society defines **complementary** medicine or methods as those that are used along with your regular medical care. If these treatments are carefully managed, they may add to your comfort and well-being. **Alternative** medicines are defined as those that are used instead of your regular medical care. Some of them have been proven not to be useful or even to be harmful, but are still promoted as "cures." If you choose to use these alternatives, they may reduce your chance of fighting your cancer by delaying, replacing, or interfering with regular cancer treatment.

Before changing your treatment or adding any of these methods, discuss this openly with your doctor or nurse. Some methods can be safely used along with standard medical treatment. Others, however, can interfere with standard treatment or cause serious side effects. That is why it's important to talk with your doctor. More information about specific complementary and alternative therapies used for cancer is available through our toll-free number or on our Web site.

Considering Prostate Cancer Treatment Options

If you have prostate cancer, there are many important factors such as your age and general health to consider before deciding on a treatment option. You should also think about which side effects you can live with. Some men, for example, can't imagine living with side effects such as incontinence or impotence. Other men are less concerned about these and more concerned about removing or destroying the cancer.

If you are over 70 or have serious health problems, you might find it useful to think of prostate cancer as a chronic disease that will probably not lead to your death but may cause symptoms you want to avoid. You may want to think more seriously about avoiding treatments that are likely to cause side effects, such as radiation and surgery, and instead consider hormone therapy or watchful waiting (careful follow-up with your doctor).

If you are in your 50s or 60s and otherwise healthy, you might be more interested in treatments that offer you the best chance for cure. Most doctors now believe that external radiation, radical prostatectomy, and brachytherapy (radioactive implants) have about the same cure rates for the earliest stage prostate cancers. The chance of being cured is influenced by factors such as your PSA level, your cancer's stage, and your Gleason score. However, the possible side effects from these forms of treatment (described above) are slightly different.

Such a complex decision is often hard to make by yourself and age itself is not necessarily the best criterion to make your choice. Many men are quite youthful at age 70 while a few, at 60, are frail and debilitated. Talk with your family and friends and consider getting more than one medical opinion. It is natural for surgical specialists such as urologists to recommend surgery and for radiation oncologists to recommend radiation. Primary care doctors can help you choose the treatment that is best for you.

You might find that speaking with others who have faced or are currently facing the same issues is useful. The American Cancer Society's program, Man to Man, and similar programs sponsored by other organizations provide a forum for you to meet and discuss these and other cancer-related issues. For more information about our programs, call us toll-free at 1-800-ACS-2345 or visit our Web site at www.cancer.org.

Treatment of Prostate Cancer by Stage

The section "How Is Prostate Cancer Staged?" explained how the T, N, and M classifications are used to stage your cancer. The stage of your cancer is one of the most important factors in deciding the best way to treat it.

What follows is a description of the treatments that may be options for men with prostate cancer diagnosed at a specific stage. But keep in mind that other factors, such as age, life expectancy, and risk of cancer recurrence after treatment (based on factors like Gleason score and PSA level) must also be considered when determining treatment options.

Stage I

These prostate cancers are small and have low Gleason scores. They usually grow very slowly and may never cause any symptoms or other health problems.

For men without any prostate cancer symptoms who are elderly and/or have other serious health problems, watchful waiting or radiation therapy (external beam or brachytherapy) are reasonable options.

Men who are younger and healthy may consider watchful waiting, radical prostatectomy, or radiation therapy (external beam or brachytherapy).

Stage II

Compared with stage I prostate cancers, stage II cancers that are not treated with surgery or radiation are more likely to eventually spread beyond the prostate and cause symptoms.

As with stage I cancers, watchful waiting by following PSA levels is often a good option for men whose cancer is not causing any symptoms and who are elderly and/or have other serious health problems. Radical prostatectomy and radiation therapy (external beam or brachytherapy) may also be appropriate options.

Treatment options for men who are younger and otherwise healthy include:

- radical prostatectomy (often with removal of the pelvic lymph nodes; sometimes preceded by hormone therapy)
- external beam radiation only*
- brachytherapy only*
- brachytherapy and external beam radiation combined*

- radical prostatectomy followed by external beam radiation if your cancer was T3 or had a high Gleason score

all the radiation options may be accompanied by 3 to 6 months of hormone therapy

Stage III

Stage III cancers have spread beyond the prostate gland but have not reached the bladder, rectum, lymph nodes, or distant organs. Curative treatments such as surgery and radiation therapy may be less likely to work but may still be options.

Treatment options at this stage may include:

- external beam radiation plus hormone therapy
- hormone therapy only
- radical prostatectomy in selected cases - not nerve sparing (often with removal of the pelvic lymph nodes; sometimes preceded by hormone therapy). This may be followed by radiation therapy.
- watchful waiting for older men whose cancer is causing no symptoms or for those who have another more serious illness

Stage IV

Stage IV cancers have already spread to the bladder, rectum, lymph nodes, or distant organs such as the bones. These cancers are generally not considered to be curable.

Treatment options may include:

- hormone therapy
- external beam radiation plus hormone therapy (in selected cases)

- surgery (TURP) to relieve symptoms such as bleeding or urinary obstruction
- watchful waiting for older men whose cancer is causing no symptoms or for those who have another serious illness

If symptoms are not relieved by standard treatments and the cancer continues to grow and spread, chemotherapy can be considered as an option. You may also want to consider taking part in a clinical trial. Treatment of stage IV prostate cancer may also include treatments for relief (palliation) of symptoms such as bone pain.

Follow-up after curative treatment

After treatment, whether radiation or surgery, your PSA level will get very low. After surgery it should be undetectable and after radiation it will drop to a very low level. Some PSA remains because the radiation didn't kill all the normal prostate cells and they will produce PSA. Your doctor will monitor your PSA levels usually every 6 months.

If your PSA level begins to rise (although it is normal for PSA to "bump" up 2 to 3 years after radiotherapy— but then it stabilizes) this means the cancer is returning. It can be coming back either at the site of your prostate or it may have spread. Your doctor will most likely order a bone scan and perhaps an MRI or CT scan of the pelvis.

Recurrent prostate cancer

If the PSA level indicates the prostate cancer has not been cured or has come back (recurred) after initial treatment, follow-up therapy will depend on where the cancer is thought to be located and what treatment(s) you have already had. (Usually, the same type of treatment is not an option. For example, men who have already had radiation therapy cannot have radiation therapy again.)

If the cancer is still thought to be localized to the area of the prostate, a second attempt at curative therapy may be possible. If you've had a radical prostatectomy, radiation therapy may be helpful. If your initial treatment was radiation, radical prostatectomy may still be an option in selected cases, although it carries a high risk for potential side effects. Cryosurgery may also be an option if the cancer is still localized.

If the cancer has spread outside the prostate gland and nearby lymph nodes the most likely site it will be found is bone. This can be detected by a bone scan. Much less often the cancer will spread to the liver or other organs. If it has spread to other parts of the body, hormone therapy is probably the most effective treatment. Radiation therapy (using external beams or radiopharmaceuticals) or other treatments (medicines such as bisphosphonates) may be given to relieve symptoms of bone pain. The hormone therapy will be given as long as the cancer is responding. This is determined by the PSA level and your own symptoms. Usually the first treatment is androgen deprivation. If this becomes ineffective, antiandrogens are used. Other hormonal agents such as diethylstilbestrol, a female hormone may be helpful and can sometimes lead to a remission of the cancer.

Remember that prostate cancer is typically slow growing, so even if it does come back, it may not be fatal. In a study of men with a PSA rise after surgery, over half the men were still alive after 15 years. Similar results were seen for men whose prostate cancer recurred after radiation therapy.

Hormone-refractory prostate cancer (HRPC)

Cancer that is no longer responding to hormone therapy such as LHRH analogs or antiandrogens is considered hormone-refractory, and can be difficult to treat. At one time it was thought that chemotherapy was not effective against prostate cancer, but in recent years this notion has been challenged. Several chemotherapy drugs have been shown to reduce PSA levels and improve quality of life. Recent studies of chemotherapy regimens that include the drug docetaxel combined with prednisone, estramustine, or both have shown that they can improve survival by several months as well as reducing pain.

Bisphosphonates appear to be helpful for many men whose cancer has spread to the bones, reducing pain and even slowing cancer growth in many cases. Other medicines and techniques are also available to keep pain and other symptoms under control. Radioactive strontium or samarium may reduce pain and even lead to a partial remission of the cancer.

If you are having pain from your prostate cancer, you should also receive pain medications from your doctor. There are many very effective drugs that can relieve pain. But, for this to happen, you must make it clear to your doctor that you have pain.

There are several promising new agents now being tested against prostate cancer, including vaccines, monoclonal antibodies, and differentiating agents.

Because our ability to treat hormone-refractory prostate cancer is still largely unsatisfactory, men are encouraged to explore these options by taking part in clinical trials.

More Treatment Information

For more details on treatment options, the National Comprehensive Cancer Network (NCCN) and the National Cancer Institute (NCI) are good sources of information.

The NCCN, made up of experts from 19 of the nation's leading cancer centers, develops cancer treatment guidelines for doctors to use when treating patients. Those are available on the NCCN Web site (www.nccn.org).

The American Cancer Society collaborates with the NCCN to produce a version of some of these treatment guidelines, written specifically for patients and their families. These less-technical versions are available on both the NCCN Web site (www.nccn.org) and the ACS Web site (www.cancer.org). A print version can also be requested from the ACS at 1-800-ACS-2345.

The NCI provides treatment guidelines via its telephone information center (1-800-4-CANCER) and its Web site (www.cancer.gov). Detailed guidelines intended for use by cancer care professionals are also available on www.cancer.gov.

Questions To Ask

What Should You Ask Your Doctor About Prostate Cancer?

It is important for you to have honest, open discussions with your cancer care team. They want to answer all of your questions, no matter how trivial you might think they are. For instance, consider asking these questions:

- ❑ What is the likelihood that the cancer has spread beyond my prostate? If so, is it still curable?
- ❑ What additional tests do you recommend, and why?
- ❑ What is the clinical stage and Gleason score (grade) of my cancer? What do those mean in my case?
- ❑ What is my expected survival rate based on clinical stage, grade, and various treatment options?
- ❑ Should I consider watchful waiting as an option? Why or why not?
- ❑ Do you recommend a radical prostatectomy or radiation? Why or why not?

- ❏ If you recommend radical prostatectomy, will it be nerve sparing? Will it be laparoscopic?
- ❏ What other treatment(s) might be appropriate for me? Why?
- ❏ Among those treatments, what are the risks or side effects that I should expect?
- ❏ What are the chances that I will have problems with incontinence or impotence?
- ❏ What are the chances that I will have other urinary or rectal problems?
- ❏ What are the chances of recurrence of my cancer with the treatment programs we have discussed?
- ❏ Should I follow a special diet?

In addition to these sample questions, be sure to write down some of your own. For instance, you might want to ask about recovery time so that you can plan your work schedule. If you are younger, you may want to discuss your plans for children if there is a possibility you could become impotent or sterile. You also may want to ask about second opinions or about clinical trials for which you may qualify.

Post-Treatment

What Happens After Treatment for Prostate Cancer?

Completing treatment can be both stressful and exciting. You will be relieved to finish treatment, yet it is hard not to worry about cancer coming back. (When cancer returns, it is called recurrence.) This is a very common concern among those who have had cancer.

It may take a while before your confidence in your own recovery begins to feel real and your fears are somewhat relieved. Even with no recurrences, people who have had cancer learn to live with uncertainty.

Follow-up Care

After treatment for prostate cancer, your doctor will want to watch you carefully, checking to see if your cancer recurs or spreads further. Your doctor should also outline a follow-up plan. This plan usually includes regular doctor visits, PSA blood tests, and digital rectal exams. Bone scans or other imaging tests may also be done, depending on your medical situation. This is the time for you to ask your health care team any questions you need answered and to discuss any concerns you might have.

Almost any cancer treatment can have side effects. Some may last for a few weeks to several months, but others can be permanent. Don't hesitate to tell your cancer care team about any symptoms or side effects that bother you so they can help you manage them.

It is also important to keep medical insurance. Even though no one wants to think of their cancer coming back, it is always a possibility. If it happens, the last thing you want is to have to worry about paying for treatment. Many people have been bankrupted by cancer recurrence.

Prostate cancer can recur many years after initial treatment, which is why it is important to keep regular doctor visits and report any new symptoms (such as bone pain or problems with urination). Should your prostate cancer come back, your treatment options will depend on where it is thought to be located and what types of treatment you've already had. For more information, see "How Is Prostate Cancer Treated?"

Seeing a New Doctor

At some point after your cancer diagnosis and treatment, you may find yourself in the office of a new doctor. Your original doctor may have moved or retired, or you may have moved or changed doctors for some reason. It is important that you be able to give your new doctor the exact details of your diagnosis and treatment. Make sure you have the following information handy:

- a copy of your pathology report from any biopsy or surgery
- if you had surgery, a copy of your operative report
- if you were hospitalized, a copy of the discharge summary that every doctor must prepare when patients are sent home from the hospital

- finally, since some drugs can have long-term side effects, a list of your drugs, drug doses, and when you took them

Lifestyle Changes to Consider During and After Treatment

Having cancer and dealing with treatment can be time-consuming and emotionally draining, but it can also be a time to look at your life in new ways. Maybe you are thinking about how to improve your health over the long term. Some people even begin this process during cancer treatment.

Make Healthier Choices

Think about your life before you learned you had cancer. Were there things you did that might have made you less healthy? Maybe you drank too much alcohol, or ate more than you needed, or smoked, or didn't exercise very often. Emotionally, maybe you kept your feelings bottled up, or maybe you let stressful situations go on too long.

Now is not the time to feel guilty or to blame yourself. However, you can start making changes today that can have positive effects for the rest of your life. Not only will you feel better but you will also be healthier. What better time than now to take advantage of the motivation you have as a result of going through a life-changing experience like having cancer?

You can start by working on those things that you feel most concerned about. Get help with those that are harder for you. For instance, if you are thinking about quitting smoking and need help, call the American Cancer Society's Quitline® tobacco cessation program at 1-800-ACS-2345.

Diet and Nutrition

Eating right can be a challenge for anyone, but it can get even tougher during and after cancer treatment. For instance, treatment often may change your sense of taste. Nausea can be a problem. You may lose your appetite for a while and lose weight when you don't want to. On the other hand, some people gain weight even without eating more. This can be frustrating, too.

If you are losing weight or have taste problems during treatment, do the best you can with eating and remember that these problems usually improve over time. You may want to ask your cancer team for a referral to a dietitian, an expert in nutrition who can give you ideas on how to fight some of the side effects of your treatment. You may also find it helps to eat small portions every 2 to 3 hours until you feel better and can go back to a more normal schedule.

One of the best things you can do after treatment is to put healthy eating habits into place. You will be surprised at the long-term benefits of some simple changes, like increasing the variety of healthy foods you eat. Try to eat 5 or more servings of vegetables and fruits each day. Choose whole grain foods instead of white flour and sugars. Try to limit meats that are high in fat. Cut back on processed meats like hot dogs, bologna, and bacon. Get rid of them altogether if you can. If you drink alcohol, limit yourself to 1 or 2 drinks a day at the most. And don't forget to get some type of regular exercise. The combination of a good diet and regular exercise will help you maintain a healthy weight and keep you feeling more energetic.

Rest, Fatigue, Work, and Exercise

Fatigue is a very common symptom in people being treated for cancer. This is often not an ordinary type of tiredness but a "bone-weary" exhaustion that doesn't get better with rest. For some, this fatigue lasts a long time after treatment, and can discourage them from physical activity.

However, exercise can actually help you reduce fatigue. Studies have shown that patients who follow an exercise program tailored to their personal needs feel physically and emotionally improved and can cope better.

If you are ill and need to be on bed rest during treatment, it is normal to expect your fitness, endurance, and muscle strength to decline some. Physical therapy can help you maintain strength and range of motion in your muscles, which can help fight fatigue and the sense of depression that sometimes comes with feeling so tired.

Any program of physical activity should fit your own situation. An older person who has never exercised will not be able to take on the same amount of exercise as a 20-year-old who plays tennis 3 times a week. If you haven't exercised in a few years but can still get around, you may want to think about taking short walks.

Talk with your health care team before starting, and get their opinion about your exercise plans. Then, try to get an exercise buddy so that you're not doing it alone. Having family or friends involved when starting a new exercise program can give you that extra boost of support to keep you going when the push just isn't there.

If you are very tired, though, you will need to balance activity with rest. It is okay to rest when you need to. It is really hard for some people to allow themselves to do that when they are used to working all day or taking care of a household. (For more information about fatigue, please see the publication, "Cancer Related Fatigue and Anemia Treatment Guidelines for Patients.")

Exercise can improve your physical and emotional health.

- It improves your cardiovascular (heart and circulation) fitness.
- It strengthens your muscles.
- It reduces fatigue.
- It lowers anxiety and depression.
- It makes you feel generally happier.
- It helps you feel better about yourself.

And long term, we know that exercise plays a role in preventing some cancers. The American Cancer Society, in its guidelines on physical activity for cancer prevention, recommends that adults take part in at least 1 physical activity for 30 minutes or more on 5 days or more of the week. Children and teens are encouraged to try for at least 60 minutes a day of energetic physical activity on at least 5 days a week.

How About Your Emotional Health?

Once your treatment ends, you may find yourself overwhelmed by emotions. This happens to a lot of people. You may have been going through so much during treatment that you could only focus on getting through your treatment.

Now you may find that you think about the potential of your own death, or the effect of your cancer on your family, friends, and career. You may also begin to re-evaluate your relationship with your spouse or partner. Unexpected issues may also cause concern—for instance, as you become healthier and have fewer doctor visits, you will see your health care team less often. That can be a source of anxiety for some.

This is an ideal time to seek out emotional and social support. You need people you can turn to for strength and comfort. Support can come in many forms: family, friends, cancer support groups, church or spiritual groups, online support communities, or individual counselors.

Almost everyone who has been through cancer can benefit from getting some type of support. What's best for you depends on your situation and personality. Some people feel safe in peer-support groups or education groups. Others would rather talk in an informal setting, such as church. Others may feel more at ease talking one-on-one with a trusted friend or counselor. Whatever your source of strength or comfort, make sure you have a place to go with your concerns.

The cancer journey can feel very lonely. It is not necessary or realistic to go it all by yourself. And your friends and family may feel shut out if you decide not to include them. Let them in—and let in anyone else who you feel may help. If you aren't sure who can help, call your American Cancer Society at 1-800-ACS-2345 and we can put you in touch with an appropriate group or resource.

You can't change the fact that you have had cancer. What you can change is how you live the rest of your life—making healthy choices and feeling as well as possible, physically and emotionally.

What Happens if Treatment Is No Longer Working?

If cancer continues to grow after one kind of treatment, or if it returns, it is often possible to try another treatment plan that might still cure the cancer, or at least shrink the tumors enough to help you live longer and feel better. On the other hand, when a person has received several different medical treatments and the cancer has not been cured, over time the cancer tends to become resistant to all treatment. At this time it's important to weigh the possible limited benefit of a new treatment against the possible downsides, including continued doctor visits and treatment side effects.

Everyone has his or her own way of looking at this. Some people may want to focus on remaining comfortable during their limited time left.

This is likely to be the most difficult time in your battle with cancer—when you have tried everything medically within reason and it's just not working anymore. Although your doctor may offer you new treatment, you need to consider that at some point, continuing treatment is not likely to improve your health or change your prognosis or survival.

If you want to continue treatment to fight your cancer as long as you can, you still need to consider the odds of more treatment having any benefit. In many cases, your doctor can estimate the response rate for the treatment you are considering. Some people are tempted to try more chemotherapy or radiation, for example, even when their doctors say that the odds of benefit are less than 1%. In this situation, you need to think about and understand your reasons for choosing this plan.

No matter what you decide to do, it is important that you be as comfortable as possible. Make sure you are asking for and getting treatment for any symptoms you might have, such as pain. This type of treatment is called **palliative treatment**.

Palliative treatment helps relieve these symptoms, but is not expected to cure the disease; its main purpose is to improve your quality of life. Sometimes, the treatments you get to control your symptoms are similar to the treatments used to treat cancer. For example, radiation therapy might be given to help relieve bone pain from bone metastasis. Or chemotherapy might be given to help shrink a tumor and keep it from causing a bowel obstruction. But this is not the same as receiving treatment to try to cure the cancer.

At some point, you may benefit from hospice care. Most of the time, this can be given at home. Your cancer may be causing symptoms or problems that need attention, and hospice focuses on your comfort. You should know that receiving hospice care doesn't mean you can't have treatment for the problems caused by your cancer or other health conditions. It just means that the focus of your care is on living life as fully as possible and feeling as well as you can at this difficult stage of your cancer.

Remember also that maintaining hope is important. Your hope for a cure may not be as bright, but there is still hope for good times with family and friends—times that are filled with happiness and meaning. In a way, pausing at this time in your cancer treatment is an opportunity to refocus on the most important things in your life. This is the time to do some things you've always wanted to do and to stop doing the things you no longer want to do.

Latest Research

What's New in Prostate Cancer Research and Treatment?

Genetics

New research on genes linked to prostate cancer is helping scientists better understand how prostate cancer develops. Further studies are expected to provide answers about the chemical changes that lead to prostate cancer. This could make it possible to design medicines to reverse those changes. Tests to find abnormal prostate cancer genes could also help identify men at high risk who would benefit from more intensive screening or from chemoprevention trials.

An exciting new development in genetics research is the use of DNA microarray technology, which allows scientists to study thousands of genes at the same time. Using this technology, researchers have identified several genes now thought to play a role in prostate cancer. This may eventually provide more sensitive screening tests for prostate cancer than the PSA blood test currently in use.

One of the biggest problems now facing patients with prostate cancer and their doctors is determining which cancers are likely to stay confined to the gland, and which are more likely to grow and spread (and therefore require treatment). The product of one gene identified by DNA microarray, known as EZH2, appears more often in advanced prostate cancers than in those at an early stage. Researchers are now trying to determine if the presence of this gene product, or others, indicates that a cancer is more aggressive. This could eventually help distinguish men who need treatment from those who might be better served by watchful waiting.

Prevention

Researchers continue to look for foods that increase or decrease prostate cancer risk. Scientists have found some substances in tomatoes (lycopenes) and soybeans (isoflavones) that may help prevent prostate cancer. Studies are underway to examine the possible effects of these compounds more closely. Scientists are also trying to develop related compounds that are even more potent and might be used as dietary supplements.

Some studies suggest that certain vitamin and mineral supplements (such as vitamin E and selenium) may lower prostate cancer risk. A large study of this issue, called the Selenium and Vitamin E Cancer Prevention Trial (SELECT), is still in progress. Another vitamin that may be important is vitamin D. Recent studies have found that men with high levels of this vitamin have a lower risk of developing the more lethal forms of prostate cancer.

Scientists are also testing using certain hormonal medicines as a way of reducing prostate cancer risk. Finasteride (Proscar) and dutasteride (Avodart) are drugs that lower the body's levels of a potent androgen called DHT. Both drugs are already used to treat benign prostatic hyperplasia (BPH). The results of one such study, the Prostate Cancer Prevention Trial, were recently reported, and are discussed in the section, "Can Prostate Cancer Be Prevented?" Although this study did not show a clear cut benefit for finasteride, a study is still in progress testing whether dutasteride might be more beneficial.

Also, scientists are learning more about the target of these drugs, a molecule called SRD5A2. This molecule is responsible for making the male hormone DHT in the prostate. Many researchers believe if they can completely shut down the activity of SRD5A2, they can block the development of prostate cancer and many compounds are being studied.

Staging

Staging plays a key role in determining which treatment options a man may be eligible for. But imaging tests for prostate cancer, such as CT and MRI scans, can't detect all cancers, especially small areas of cancer in lymph nodes. A newer technique, called **enhanced MRI**, may help find lymph nodes that contain cancer. Patients first undergo a standard MRI. They are then injected with tiny magnetic particles, and have another scan done the next day. Differences between the 2 scans point to possible cancer cells in the lymph nodes. Early results of this technique are promising, but it will need more study before it becomes widely used.

Treatment

Surgery

If the nerves that control erections (which run along either side of the prostate) must be removed during the operation, a man will become impotent. Some doctors are now exploring the use of sural nerve grafts to try to restore potency if the original nerves must be removed. This approach, done at the same time as the radical prostatectomy, involves replacing the original nerves with small nerves taken from the side of the foot. This is still considered an experimental technique, and not all doctors agree as to its usefulness. Further study is underway.

Radiation therapy

As described in the section, "How Is Prostate Cancer Treated?" advances in technology are making it possible to aim radiation more precisely than in the past. Currently used techniques such as conformal radiation therapy (CRT) and intensity modulated radiation therapy (IMRT) allow doctors to treat only the prostate gland and to try as much as possible to avoid radiation to normal tissues. This is expected to increase the effectiveness and reduce the side effects of radiation therapy. Studies are underway to find out which radiation techniques are best suited for specific categories of patients with prostate cancer.

Technology is making other forms of radiation therapy more effective as well. New computer programs allow doctors to better plan the radiation doses and approaches for both external radiation therapy and brachytherapy. Planning for brachytherapy can now even be done during the procedure (intraoperatively).

Newer treatments for localized disease

Researchers are now studying newer forms of treatment for early stage prostate cancer, either as primary treatment or to be used after radiation therapy if it was not thought to be successful.

Chemotherapy

Studies in recent years have shown that many chemotherapy drugs can affect prostate cancer, and at least one has been shown to help men live longer. Several new chemotherapy drugs and combinations of drugs are now being studied.

Calcitriol, a form of vitamin D, has recently shown promising results when combined with the chemotherapy drug docetaxel (Taxotere). Men who received the combination seemed to do better than men in other studies who received only docetaxel. A large clinical trial is now underway to compare treatment with the combination of calcitriol and docetaxel with treatment with docetaxel alone. Phenoxodiol is another vitamin-like drug that is being tested in men with advanced prostate cancer.

Prostate cancer vaccine therapy

Several types of vaccines for boosting the body's immune response to prostate cancer cells are being tested in clinical trials. One technique removes dendritic cells (cells of the immune system) from the patient's blood and exposes them to a component of prostate cancer cells called prostate-specific membrane antigen (PSMA). These cells are then put back into the body, where they induce other immune system cells to attack the patient's prostate cancer. A recent report stated that a vaccine called Provenge increased survival in men with widespread prostate cancer. Several other vaccines are also being tested in clinical trials. At this time, vaccines are only available in clinical trials. Provenge has been submitted to the FDA for approval.

Other prostate cancer vaccines use genetically modified viruses that contain prostate-specific antigen (PSA). The patient is injected with the virus. His immune system responds to the virus and also becomes sensitized to cancer cells containing PSA and destroys these cells.

Monoclonal antibodies

These are antibodies made in the laboratory that target specific molecules in the prostate cancer cell. Several different ones are being developed and tested. They act by either killing the cells by stimulating the body's natural cell-killing mechanism or they can carry a radioactive molecule that can kill the cell. One such antibody directed against prostate cancer cells has been developed. It contains a radioactive molecule, lutenium, and has shown some benefit in early trials.

Endothelin inhibitors

Endothelin A is a naturally occurring substance that helps prostate cancer cells to grow. A new drug, called atrasentan (Xinlay), can block the effects of endothelin A. When given to men with advanced prostate cancer it slowed progression of their cancer and relieved symptoms. It was rejected for approval by the FDA until further clinical trials are completed. Other endothelin inhibitors are in clinical trials and one of these my receive FDA approval in the near future.

Angiogenesis inhibitors

Growth of prostate cancer depends on growth of blood vessels (**angiogenesis**) to nourish the cancer cells. Analysis of angiogenesis in prostate cancer specimens can help predict prognosis. Cancers that stimulate many new vessels to grow have a poorer outlook. New drugs are being studied that may be useful in stopping prostate cancer growth by keeping new blood vessels from forming.

Several antiangiogenic drugs are already being tested in clinical trials. One of these is thalidomide, which has been approved by the FDA and is used to treat patients with multiple myeloma. It is being combined with chemotherapy in clinical trials to treat men with advanced prostate cancer. It causes major side effects of constipation, drowsiness and nerve damage. Newer versions of the drug with fewer side effects have been developed. A second drug is called bevacizumab. This is also an FDA-approved drug that is used to treat patients with advanced colorectal cancer. It is being tested in men with advanced prostate cancer, mainly in combination with chemotherapy.

Targeted therapy

Many new anti-cancer drugs have been developed that attach to certain substances in the cancer cell and kill the cell. Work is now ongoing in developing similar agents for prostate cancer. One likely target is the androgen receptor—the molecule that takes its growth cue from testosterone.

Treatment of bone pain

Doctors are now studying the use of radiofrequency ablation (RFA) to help control pain in men whose prostate cancer has spread to one or more areas in the bones. During RFA, the doctor uses computed tomography (CT) or ultrasound to guide a small metal probe into the area of the tumor. A high frequency current passed through the probe heats and destroys the tumor. While RFA has been used for many years to treat tumors in other organs such as the liver, its use in treating bone pain is still relatively new.

Nutrition and lifestyle changes

A recent report found that men who decided not to have treatment for their localized prostate cancer may be able to slow its growth with intensive lifestyle changes. The men ate a vegan (no meat, fish, eggs, or dairy products) diet and exercised. They also participated in support groups and yoga. After one year, the men saw, on average, a slight drop in their PSA level. It isn't known whether this effect will last since the report only followed the men for one year.

Resources

Additional Resources

More Information From Your American Cancer Society

We have selected some related information that may also be helpful to you. These materials may be viewed on our Web site or ordered from our toll-free number, 1-800-ACS-2345.

Caring for the Patient With Cancer at Home: A Guide for Patients and Families (also available in Spanish)

Guidelines for the Early Detection of Cancer (also available in Spanish)

Managing Incontinence After Treatment For Prostate Cancer

Prostate Cancer: Treatment Guidelines for Patients – Version V (also available in Spanish)

Sexuality and Cancer: For the Man Who Has Cancer and His Partner (also available in Spanish)

The following books are available from the American Cancer Society. Call us at 1-800-ACS-2345 to ask about costs or to place your order.

American Cancer Society's Consumer Guide to Cancer Drugs, Second Edition

American Cancer Society's Complete Guide to Prostate Cancer

*American Cancer Society's Guide to Pain Control:
Understanding and Managing Cancer Pain,*
Revised Edition

Because… Someone I Love Has Cancer: Kids' Activity Book

*Cancer in the Family: Helping Children Cope with a
Parent's Illness*

*Caregiving: A Step-By-Step Resource for Caring for the
Person With Cancer at Home,* Revised Edition

*Coming to Terms With Cancer: A Glossary of Cancer-
Related Terms*

*Couples Confronting Cancer: Keeping Your
Relationship Strong*

Eating Well, Staying Well During and After Cancer

*Informed Decisions: The Complete Book of Cancer
Diagnosis, Treatment, and Recovery,* Second Edition

*Lymphedema: Understanding and Managing Lymphedema
After Cancer Treatment*

National Organizations and Web Sites*

In addition to the American Cancer Society, other sources of patient information and support include:

American Urological Association
Telephone: 1-800-828-7866;
1-800-242-2383 (for ordering materials only)
Internet Address: www.auanet.org

National Association for Continence
Telephone: 1-800-252-3337 (1-800-BLADDER)
Internet Address: www.nafc.org

National Cancer Institute
Telephone: 1-800-422-6237 (1-800-4-CANCER);
TYY: 1-800-332-8615
Internet Address: www.cancer.gov

National Coalition for Cancer Survivorship
Telephone: 1-877-622-7937 (1-877-NCCS-YES)
Internet Address: www.canceradvocacy.org

National Comprehensive Cancer Network
Internet Address: www.nccn.org

National Prostate Cancer Coalition
Telephone: 1-888-245-9455
Internet Address: www.pcacoalition.org

Prostate Cancer Foundation (formerly "CaP Cure")
Telephone: 1-800-757-2873 (1-800-757-CURE)
or 1-310-570-4700
Internet Address: www.prostatecancerfoundation.org

US Too International, Inc.
Telephone: 1-800-808-7866 (1-800-80US TOO)
or 1-630-795-1002 (Chicago area)
Internet Address: www.ustoo.com

Inclusion on this list does not imply endorsement by the American Cancer Society

The American Cancer Society is happy to address almost any cancer-related topic. If you have any more questions, please call us at 1-800-ACS-2345 any time, 24 hours a day.

References

American Cancer Society. *Cancer Facts and Figures 2006*. Atlanta, Ga: American Cancer Society; 2006.

American Joint Committee on Cancer. Prostate. In: *AJCC Cancer Staging Manual*. 6th ed. New York, NY: Springer; 2002:309-316.

Hellerstedt BA, Pienta KJ. The current state of hormonal therapy for prostate cancer. *CA Cancer J Clin*. 2002;52:154-179.

National Comprehensive Cancer Network. *Clinical Practice Guidelines in Oncology: Prostate Cancer.* Available at: www.nccn.org. Accessed Jan 2006.

Oh WK, Hurwitz M, D'Amico AV, Richie JP, Kantoff PW. Neoplasms of the prostate. In: Kufe DW, Pollock RE, Weichselbaum RR, Bast RC, Gansler TS, Holland JF, Frei E III, eds. *Cancer Medicine*. Hamilton, Ontario: BC Decker; 2003:1707-1740.

Potosky AL, Davis WW, Hoffman RM. Five-year outcomes after prostatectomy or radiotherapy for prostate cancer: The prostate cancer outcomes study. *J Natl Cancer Inst*. 2004;96:1358-1367.

Prostate Cancer Foundation. *Report to the Nation on Prostate Cancer 2004*. Available at: www.prostatecancerfoundation.org. Accessed Feb 2005.

Scher HI, Leibel SA, Fuks ZY, Cordona-Cardo C. Scardino PT. Cancer of the prostate. In: DeVita VT, Hellman S, Rosenberg SA, eds. *Cancer: Principles and Practice of Oncology*. Philadelphia, Pa: Lippincott-Raven; 2005:1192-1259.

Smith, RA, Cokkinides V, Eyre HJ. American Cancer Society guidelines for the early detection of cancer, 2004. *CA Cancer J Clin*. 2004;54:41-52.

Dictionary

PROSTATE CANCER DICTIONARY

3DCRT: see three-dimensional conformal radiation therapy.

5-alpha reductase: an enzyme that converts testosterone to a more active hormone called dihydrotestosterone (DHT). Drugs such a finasteride (Proscar or Propecia) that prevent this conversion are called 5-alpha reductase inhibitors and may help reduce the risk of prostate cancer.

ablative therapy: treatment that removes or destroys the function of an organ; for example, removing the ovaries or testicles or having some types of treatment that cause them to stop working.

adenocarcinoma: cancer that starts in the glandular tissue, such as the prostate.

adrenal glands: small glands located on top of each kidney. Their main function is to produce hormones that control metabolism, fluid balance, and blood pressure. In addition, they produce small amounts of "male" hormones (androgens) and "female" hormones (estrogens and progesterone).

adjuvant therapy: treatment used in addition to the main treatment. It usually refers to hormonal therapy, chemotherapy, or radiation added after primary treatment to increase the chances of curing the disease or keeping it in check.

advanced cancer: general term describing stages of cancer in which the disease has spread from the primary site to other parts of the body. When the cancer has spread only to the surrounding areas, it is called locally advanced. If it has spread to distant parts of the body, it is called metastatic.

advance directives: legal documents that tell the doctor and family what a person wants for future medical care, including whether to start or when to stop life-sustaining treatment.

alopecia: hair loss. This often occurs as a result of chemotherapy or from radiation therapy to the head. In most cases, the hair grows back after treatment ends.

alpha blocker: a drug that relaxes smooth muscle tissue. Alpha blockers are sometimes used to help men who have difficulty urinating due to benign prostatic hyperplasia (BPH) or other causes.

alternative therapy: use of an unproven therapy instead of standard (proven) therapy. Some alternative therapies may have dangerous or even life-threatening side effects. For others, the main danger is that a patient may lose the opportunity to benefit from standard therapy. The ACS recommends that patients considering use of any alternative or complementary therapy discuss this with their health care team. *See also* complementary therapy.

analog: a manmade version of a naturally occurring substance. *See also* LHRH analog.

anastomosis: the site where two structures are surgically joined together, such as the bladder neck and the urethra after removal of the prostate.

androgen: any male sex hormone. The major androgen is testosterone.

androgen ablation: *see* combination hormone therapy.

androgen blockade: use of drugs to disrupt the actions of male hormones.

androgen-dependent: term used to describe prostate cells, benign or malignant, that are stimulated to grow and multiply by male hormones and are suppressed by drugs that disrupt the action of male hormones.

androgen deprivation therapy (ADT): *see* hormone therapy

androgen-independent: term for prostate cancer cells that no longer respond to hormone therapy; also known as hormone-refractory.

anesthesia: the loss of feeling or sensation as a result of drugs or gases. General anesthesia causes loss of consciousness (makes you go into a deep sleep). Local or regional anesthesia numbs only a certain area of the body.

angiogenesis: the formation of new blood vessels. Some cancer treatments work by blocking angiogenesis, thus preventing blood from reaching the tumor.

antiandrogens: drugs that block the body's ability to use androgens. They are taken as pills, once or three times a day. Antiandrogens are usually used in combination with orchiectomy or LHRH analogs. Several drugs of this type are currently available—flutamide (Eulexin), bicalutamide (Casodex), and nilutamide (Nilandron).

antibody: a protein produced by the body's immune system cells and released into the blood. Antibodies defend the body against foreign agents, such as bacteria. These agents contain certain substances called antigens. Each antibody works against a specific antigen. *See also* antigen.

antiemetic: a drug that prevents or relieves nausea and vomiting, common side effects of chemotherapy.

antigen: a substance that causes the body's immune system to react, often resulting in the production of antibodies. For example, the immune system's response to antigens that are part of bacteria and viruses helps people resist infections. Cancer cells have certain antigens that can be found by laboratory tests. They are important in cancer diagnosis and in watching response to treatment. Other cancer cell antigens play a role in immune reactions that may help the body's resistance against cancer.

antioxidants: molecules such as some vitamins that block the actions of activated oxygen molecules, known as free radicals, that can damage cells.

anus: the end of the digestive tract, through which waste passes out of the body.

artificial sphincter: an inflatable cuff implanted around the upper urethra to squeeze the urethra shut and provide urinary control.

aspiration: the process of drawing out by suction. *See also* fine needle aspiration.

atypical: not usual; abnormal. Often refers to the appearance of cancerous or precancerous cells. *See also* hyperplasia.

BPH: *see* benign prostatic hyperplasia.

benign: not cancer; not malignant.

benign prostatic hyperplasia: non-cancerous enlargement of the prostate that may cause problems with urination such as trouble starting and stopping the flow. Also referred to as BPH.

biochemical failure: a term sometimes used by doctors to describe a significant rise in PSA after primary therapy which likely indicates that cancer has recurred. There may be several years, however, between a rise in PSA and when the cancer is detectable by other means.

biopsy: the removal of a sample of tissue to see whether cancer cells are present. There are several kinds of biopsies. In a fine needle aspiration biopsy (sometimes used to check pelvic lymph nodes), a very thin needle is used to draw out fluid and cells. In a core biopsy, a larger needle is used to remove a thin cylinder of tissue. *See also* sextant biopsy.

bisphosphonates: drugs that slow down the action of bone-eating cells called osteoclasts, thereby slowing the spread of cancer in the bones. Bisphosphonates are most commonly used in breast cancer and multiple myeloma (a type of bone cancer), but are now approved for use in men with prostate cancer that has spread to the bones.

bladder: a hollow organ with flexible, muscular walls that stores urine.

bone scan: an imaging test that gives important information about the bones, including the location of cancer that may have spread to the bones. It can be done on an outpatient basis and is painless, except for the needle stick when a low-dose radioactive substance is injected into a vein. Pictures are taken to see where the radioactivity collects, pointing to an abnormality.

brachytherapy: internal radiation treatment given by placing radioactive material directly into the tumor or close to it. Also called interstitial radiation therapy or seed implantation.

CAB: combined androgen blockade. *See* combination hormonal therapy.

CAT scan: *see* computed tomography

cGy: *see* centigray

CT scan: *see* computed tomography

cancer: cancer is not just one disease but rather a group of diseases. All forms of cancer cause cells in the body to change and grow out of control. Most types of cancer cells form a lump or mass called a tumor. The tumor can invade and destroy healthy tissue. Cells from the tumor can break away and travel to other parts of the body. There they can continue to grow. This spreading process is called metastasis. When cancer spreads, it is still named after the part of the body where it started. For example, if prostate cancer spreads to the bones, it is still prostate cancer, not bone cancer.

Some cancers, such as blood cancers, do not form a tumor. Not all tumors are cancer. A tumor that is not cancer is called **benign**. Benign tumors do not grow and spread the way cancer does. They are usually not a threat to life. Another word for cancerous is malignant.

cancer care team: the group of health care professionals who work together to find, treat, and care for people with cancer. The cancer care team may include any or all of the following and others: primary care physicians, pathologists, oncology specialists (medical oncologist, radiation oncologist), surgeons (including surgical specialists such as urologists, gynecologists, neurosurgeons, etc.), nurses, oncology nurse specialists, and oncology social workers. Whether the team is linked formally or informally, there is usually one person who takes the job of coordinating the team.

cancer cell: a cell that divides and reproduces abnormally and can spread throughout the body. *See also* metastasis.

cancer-related checkup: a routine health examination for cancer in persons without obvious signs or symptoms of cancer. The goal of the cancer-related checkup is to find the disease, if it exists, at an early stage, when chances for cure are greatest. Depending on the person's sex and age, this checkup could include a digital rectal examination, testicular examinations, PSA blood test, and/or skin examinations. *See also* detection.

carcinogen: any substance that causes cancer or helps cancer grow. For example, tobacco smoke contains many carcinogens that greatly increase the risk of lung cancer.

carcinoma: a malignant tumor that begins in the lining layer (epithelial cells) of organs. At least 80% of all cancers are carcinomas. Almost all prostate cancers are carcinomas, specifically adenocarcinomas.

castration: surgery to remove the testicles; the medical term is orchiectomy.

catheter (urinary): a thin, flexible tube through which fluids enter or leave the body; for example, a tube inserted through the tip of the penis into the bladder to drain urine (known as a "Foley catheter").

cell: the basic unit of which all living things are made. Cells replace themselves by splitting and forming new cells (mitosis). The processes that control the formation of new cells and the death of old cells are disrupted in cancer.

centigray (cGy): a unit of radiation equal to the older unit, the rad.

chemical castration: the use of hormone therapy medications to achieve very low levels of testosterone without surgical removal of the testicles.

chemotherapy: treatment with drugs to destroy cancer cells. Chemotherapy is often used with surgery or radiation to treat cancer when the cancer has spread, when it has come back (recurred), or when there is a strong chance that it could recur.

clinical trials: research studies to test new drugs or other treatments to compare current, standard treatments with others that may be better. Before a new treatment is used on people, it is studied in the lab. If lab studies suggest the treatment will work, the next step is to test its value for patients. These human studies are called clinical trials. The main questions the researchers want to answer are:
- Does this treatment work?
- Does it work better than what we're now using?
- What side effects does it cause?
- Do the benefits outweigh the risks?
- Which patients are most likely to find this treatment helpful?

combination hormone therapy: complete blockage of androgen production that may include castration (orchiectomy) or LHRH analogs, plus the use of antiandrogens; also called combined androgen blockade (CAB), total hormonal ablation, total androgen blockade, or total androgen ablation.

combined androgen blockade (CAB): *see* combination hormone therapy.

complementary therapy: therapy used in addition to standard therapy. Some complementary therapies may help relieve certain symptoms of cancer, relieve side effects of standard cancer therapy, or improve a patient's sense of well-being. The ACS recommends that patients considering use of any alternative or complementary therapy discuss this with their health care team. *See also* alternative therapy.

computed tomography (CT): an imaging test in which many x-ray images are taken from different angles of a part of the body. These images are combined by a computer to produce cross-sectional pictures of internal organs. Except for the injection of a dye (needed in some but not all cases), this is a painless procedure that can be done in an outpatient clinic. It is often referred to as a "CT" or "CAT" scan.

conformal proton beam radiation therapy: a technique that uses proton beams instead of conventional radiation. Protons are parts of atoms that cause little damage to tissues they pass through but are very effective in killing cells at the end of their path. This means that proton beam radiation may be able to deliver more radiation to the cancer while reducing side effects of nearby normal tissues.

corpora cavernosa and **corpus spongiosum:** chambers in the penis that fill with blood during erection.

cryoablation: use of extreme cold to freeze the prostate and destroy cancer cells. Also known as cryosurgery.

cryosurgery: *see* cryoablation.

curative treatment: treatment aimed at producing a cure. Compare with palliative treatment.

cystoscope: a slender tube with a lens and a light. It is placed into the bladder through the urethra, allowing the doctor to view the inside of these organs.

cystoscopy: examination of the bladder with an instrument called a cystoscope.

cytology: the branch of science that deals with the structure and function of cells. Also refers to tests to diagnose cancer and other diseases by examination of cells under the microscope.

cytotoxic: toxic to cells; cell-killing.

DHT (dihydrotestosterone): powerful form of male hormone produced by the action of 5-alpha reductase (a prostate enzyme) on testosterone.

DNA (deoxyribonucleic acid): the genetic "blueprint" found in the nucleus of each cell. DNA holds genetic information on cell growth, division, and function.

DRE: *see* digital rectal examination.

debulk: to surgically reduce the volume of cancer.

depot injection: an injection of a drug in a formulation that allows it to enter the bloodstream over time. LHRH analogs such as Lupron and Zoladex are depot injections, meaning that they only have to be given once a month (or once every several months).

detection: finding disease. Early detection means that the disease is found at an early stage, before it has grown large or spread to other sites. Note: many forms of cancer can reach an advanced stage without causing symptoms. The PSA blood test may help find early prostate cancer.

diagnosis: identification of a disease by its signs or symptoms and through the use of imaging procedures and laboratory findings. For some types of cancer, the earlier a diagnosis is made, the better the chance for long-term survival.

dietary supplement: a product, such as a vitamin, mineral, or herb, intended to improve health but not to diagnose, treat, cure, or prevent disease. Because dietary supplements are not considered "drugs," their manufacturers do not have to prove they are effective, or even safe.

differentiation: the normal process through which cells mature so they can carry out the jobs they were meant to do. Cancer cells are less differentiated than normal cells. Pathologists use grading to evaluate and report the degree of a cancer's differentiation.

digital rectal examination (DRE): an exam during which the doctor inserts a lubricated, gloved finger into the rectum to feel for anything not normal. Some tumors of the rectum and prostate gland can be felt during a DRE.

disease-free survival rate: the percentage of people with a certain cancer who still have no evidence of disease (cancer) a certain period of time (usually 5 years) after treatment. This rate does not measure actual "survival," which is expressed by the five-year survival rate.

doubling time: for cancer in general, the time it takes for a cell to divide and double itself. Cancers vary in doubling time from 8 to 600 days, averaging 100 to 120 days. Thus, a cancer may be present for many years before it can be felt. Compare to PSA doubling time.

ejaculate: to release semen during orgasm; as a noun, ejaculation.

epidemiology: the study of diseases in populations by collecting and analyzing statistical data. In the field of cancer, epidemiologists look at how many people have cancer; who gets specific types of cancer; and what factors (such as job hazards, family patterns, personal habits such as smoking and diet, and environment) play a part in the development of cancer.

epididymis: tiny tubes within the scrotum but outside the testicles through which sperm travel after forming and where they are stored until they mature; they lead into the vas deferens.

epidural anesthesia: injection of anesthetic drugs into the space around the spinal cord. Used to numb the lower part of the body while allowing the patient to remain awake.

erectile dysfunction: not being able to have or keep an erection of the penis; impotence.

estrogen: a female sex hormone produced primarily by the ovaries, and in smaller amounts by the adrenal cortex. It is sometimes given to men with advanced prostate cancer to counteract the action of testosterone.

etiology: the cause of a disease. There are many causes of cancer, and research is showing that both genetics and lifestyle are major factors in many cancers.

expectant management: *see* watchful waiting.

external beam radiation therapy (EBRT): radiation that is focused from a source outside the body on the area affected by the cancer. It is much like getting a diagnostic x-ray, but for a longer time and at a higher dose.

false negative: test result implying a condition does not exist when in fact it does.

false positive: test result implying a condition exists when in fact it does not.

fine needle aspiration (FNA) biopsy: a procedure in which a thin needle is used to draw up (aspirate) samples for examination under a microscope. *See also* biopsy.

first-degree relative: a parent, sibling (brother or sister), or child.

five-year survival rate: the percentage of people with a given cancer who are expected to survive 5 years or longer with the disease. Five-year survival rates have some drawbacks. Although the rates are based on the most recent information available, they may include data from patients treated several years earlier. Advances in cancer treatment often occur quickly. Five-year survival rates, while statistically valid, may not reflect these advances. They should not be seen as a predictor in an individual case. *See also* relative five-year survival rate.

free-PSA ratio: a test that indicates how much PSA circulates unbound (alone) in the blood compared to the total amount of PSA. For total PSA results in the borderline range (4 to 10 ng/mL), a low percent free-PSA (25% or less) means that a prostate cancer is more likely to be present and may suggest the need for a biopsy. Also known as percent-free PSA.

frequency, urinary: the need to urinate often.

frozen section: a very thin slice of tissue that has been quick-frozen and then examined under a microscope. This method is sometimes used during an operation because it gives a quick diagnosis, and can tell a surgeon whether or not to continue with the procedure. The diagnosis is confirmed in a few days by a more detailed study called a permanent section.

gene: a segment of DNA that contains information on hereditary characteristics such as hair color, eye color, and height, as well as susceptibility to certain diseases.

gland: a cell or group of cells that produce and release substances used nearby or in another part of the body. The prostate is an example of a gland.

glans: the head of the penis.

Gleason grade: the most often used prostate cancer grading system is called the Gleason system. A pathologist assigns a Gleason grade ranging from 1 through 5 based on how much the cancer cells under the microscope look like normal prostate cells. Those that look a lot like normal cells are graded as 1, while those that look the least like normal cells are graded as 5. *See also* Gleason score; grade.

Gleason score: the combination of the two Gleason grades used in classifying each prostate cancer, based on how the cells appear under the microscope. Because prostate cancers often have areas with different grades, a grade is assigned to the two areas that make up most of the cancer. These two grades are added together to give a Gleason score between 2 and 10. The higher the Gleason score, the faster the cancer is likely to grow and the more likely it is to spread beyond the prostate. Also known as the Gleason sum.

grade: the grade of a cancer reflects how abnormal it looks under the microscope. There are several grading systems for different types of cancers, such as the Gleason grades for prostate cancer. Each grading system divides cancer into those with the greatest abnormality, the least abnormality, and those in between.

Grading is done by a pathologist, who examines tissue from the biopsy. Cancers with more abnormal-appearing cells tend to grow and spread more quickly and have a worse prognosis (outlook).

gynecomastia: male breast enlargement, sometimes involving breast tenderness; a possible side effect of some hormone therapy.

HDR brachytherapy: see high-dose rate brachytherapy.

HER2: oncogene that may become "turned on" (activated) in some cases of prostate cancer. Activation can cause normal cells to change into cancer cells and can cause some cancer cells to grow and spread especially fast. *See also* oncogene.

HPC1: a gene linked to some cases of prostate cancer. Inherited DNA changes in HPC1 may make prostate cancer more likely to develop in some men. These changes appear to be responsible for about 10% of prostate cancers. Research on this gene is still preliminary, and a genetic test is not yet available.

hesitancy: inability to start the stream of urine promptly.

high-dose rate (HDR) brachytherapy: a form of treatment involving insertion of small plastic catheters into the prostate gland, guided by transrectal ultrasound (TRUS). A radioactive source (iridium-192) is then placed in the catheters and is removed a short time later. It is usually given once a week for 2 or 3 weeks and is often used in combination with external beam radiation. Unlike standard brachytherapy (which uses lower doses of radiation over a longer period of time) the radioactive seeds are not left in the body.

hormone: a chemical substance released into the body by the endocrine glands such as the thyroid, adrenals, or ovaries. The substance travels through the bloodstream and sets in motion various body functions. Testosterone and estrogen are examples of male and female hormones.

hormone-dependent: *see* androgen-dependent.

hormone-refractory: *see* androgen-independent.

hormone therapy: treatment with hormones, using drugs that interfere with hormone production or hormone action, or the surgical removal of hormone-producing glands. Hormone therapy may kill cancer cells or slow their growth. It is a common form of treatment for advanced prostate cancer.

hot flash: sudden rush of body heat causing reddening and sweating; a common side effect of some types of hormone therapy.

hyperplasia: too much growth of cells or tissue in a specific area, such as the lining of the prostate. Hyperplasia is not cancer, however. *See also,* benign prostatic hyperplasia.

IGF-1: *see* insulin-like growth factor-1.

IMRT: *see* intensity modulated radiation therapy

imaging studies: methods used to produce a picture of internal body structures. Some imaging methods used to help diagnose or stage cancer are x-rays, bone scans, CT scans, magnetic resonance imaging (MRI), and ultrasound.

immune system: the complex system by which the body resists infection by germs such as bacteria or viruses and rejects transplanted tissues or organs. The immune system may also help the body fight some cancers.

impotence: not being able to have or maintain an erection of the penis; erectile dysfunction.

incidence: the number of new cases of a disease that occur in a population each year. Compare to prevalence.

incision: cut made during surgery.

incontinence, urinary: partial or complete loss of urinary control. See also stress incontinence, urge incontinence, overflow incontinence.

insulin-like growth factor-1 (IGF-1): hormone-like substance thought to affect growth hormone activity. Researchers have recently noted that men with high blood levels of IGF-1may be more likely to develop prostate cancer.

intensity modulated radiation therapy (IMRT): an advanced method of conformal radiation therapy in which the beams are aimed from several directions and the intensity (strength) of the beams is controlled by computers. This allows more radiation to reach the treatment area while reducing the radiation to healthy tissues. *See also* three-dimensional conformal radiation therapy.

intermittent hormone therapy: a type of prostate cancer treatment in which hormonal drugs are stopped after a man's blood PSA level drops to a very low level and remains stable for a while. If the PSA level begins to rise, the drugs are started again.

internal radiation: treatment involving implantation of a radioactive substance into the body; see also brachytherapy.

interstitial radiation therapy: a type of internal radiation or brachytherapy treatment in which a radioactive implant is placed directly into the tissue (not in a body cavity).

intramuscular (IM): injected into a muscle.

intravenous (IV): a method of supplying fluids or medications using a needle inserted in a vein.

intravenous pyelogram (IVP): a special kind of x-ray procedure. A dye injected into the bloodstream travels to the kidneys, ureters and bladder and helps to clearly outline these organs on x-rays.

invasive cancer: cancer that has spread beyond the layer of cells where it first developed to involve adjacent tissues.

investigational: under study; often used to describe drugs used in clinical trials that are not yet available to the general public.

Kegel exercises: exercises to strengthen bladder muscles. These exercises may help men and women with certain forms of incontinence.

LH: *see* luteinizing hormone

LHRH: *see* luteinizing hormone-releasing hormone.

LHRH agonists: *see* LHRH analogs.

LHRH analogs: manmade hormones, chemically similar to LHRH. They block the production of the male hormone testosterone and are sometimes used as a treatment for prostate cancer. LHRH analogs approved for use in the US include leuprolide, goserelin, and triptorelin.

laparoscope: a long, slender tube inserted into the abdomen through a very small incision. The laparoscope allows the surgeon to view organs and lymph nodes within the body. The lymph nodes, or even the prostate gland itself, can be removed using special surgical instruments operated through the laparoscope.

laparoscopic lymphadenectomy: removal of lymph nodes with a laparoscope.

laparoscopic radical prostatectomy (LRP): a surgical procedure in which the prostate is removed using a laparoscope. This procedure is still widely considered to be experimental at this time.

libido: sex drive.

local anesthesia: *see* anesthesia.

local recurrence: *see* recurrence.

localized prostate cancer: cancer that is confined to the prostate gland.

luteinizing hormone (LH): pituitary hormone that stimulates the testicles to produce testosterone.

luteinizing hormone-releasing hormone (LHRH): a hormone produced by the hypothalamus, a tiny gland in the brain, that affects levels of LH in the body and therefore affects testosterone levels.

lycopenes: vitamin-like antioxidants that help prevent damage to DNA and may help lower prostate cancer risk. These substances are found in tomatoes, pink grapefruit, and watermelon.

lymphadenectomy: surgical removal of lymph nodes. After removal, the lymph nodes are examined by microscope to see if cancer has spread; also called lymph node dissection. *See also* lymphatic system.

lymphatic system: the tissues and organs (including lymph nodes, spleen, thymus, and bone marrow) that produce and store lymphocytes (cells that fight infection) and the channels that carry the lymph fluid. The entire lymphatic system is an important part of the body's immune system. Invasive cancers such as prostate cancer sometimes penetrate the lymphatic vessels (channels) and spread (metastasize) to lymph nodes.

> **lymph:** clear fluid that flows through the lymphatic vessels and contains cells known as lymphocytes. These cells are important in fighting infections and may also have a role in fighting cancer.

> **lymph nodes:** small bean-shaped collections of immune system tissue, such as lymphocytes, found along lymphatic vessels. They remove cell waste and fluids from lymph. They help fight infections and also have a role in fighting cancer, although cancers sometimes spread through them. Also called lymph glands.

> **lymphocyte:** a type of white blood cell that helps the body fight infection.

magnetic resonance imaging (MRI): a method of taking pictures of the inside of the body. Instead of using x-rays, MRI uses a powerful magnet to send radio waves through the body; the images appear on a computer screen as well as on film. Like x-rays, the procedure is physically painless, but some people may feel confined inside the MRI machine.

malignant tumor: a mass of cancer cells that may invade surrounding tissues or spread (metastasize) to distant areas of the body.

Man to Man: American Cancer Society program of education and support for men with prostate cancer. Call 1-800-ACS-2345 to ask about program locations.

margin, surgical: edge of the tissue removed during surgery. A negative surgical margin is a sign that no cancer was left behind. A positive surgical margin indicates that cancer cells are found at the outer edge of the tissue removed and is usually a sign that some cancer remains in the body.

medical oncologist: a doctor who is specially trained to diagnose cancer and treat cancer with chemotherapy and other drugs.

metastasis: the spread of cancer cells to distant areas of the body by way of the lymph system or bloodstream.

MRI: *see* magnetic resonance imaging

negative margin: *see* margin, surgical.

neoadjuvant therapy: treatment given before radiation or surgery. For example, neoadjuvant hormonal therapy is sometimes used to shrink the prostate tumor prior to brachytherapy to make it more effective.

neoplasm: an abnormal growth (tumor) that starts from a single altered cell; a neoplasm may be benign or malignant. Cancer is a malignant neoplasm.

nerve sparing prostatectomy: radical prostatectomy in which the surgeon attempts to maintain potency by leaving in the neurovascular bundles that control erection.

neurovascular bundle: one of two groups of nerves and blood vessels that run alongside the prostate and help the penis become erect. Removal or injury of these bundles during surgery, or damage from radiation therapy, can lead to impotence.

nocturia: frequent nighttime urination.

node: lymph node; *see* lymphatic system.

nodal status: indicates whether the cancer has spread (node-positive) or has not spread (node-negative) to lymph nodes.

nurse practitioner: a registered nurse with a master's or doctoral degree. Licensed nurse practitioners diagnose and manage illness and disease, usually working closely with a doctor. In many states, they may prescribe medications.

oncogenes: genes that promote cell growth and multiplication. These genes are normally present in all cells. But oncogenes may undergo changes that activate them, causing cells to grow too quickly and form tumors.

oncologist: a doctor with special training in the diagnosis and treatment of cancer.

oncology: the branch of medicine concerned with the diagnosis and treatment of cancer.

oncology clinical nurse specialist: a registered nurse with a master's degree in oncology who specializes in the care of cancer patients. Oncology nurse specialists may prepare and administer treatments, monitor patients, prescribe and provide supportive care, and teach and counsel patients and their families.

oncology social worker: a person with a master's degree in social work who is an expert in coordinating and providing non-medical care to patients. The oncology social worker provides counseling and assistance to people with cancer and their families, especially in dealing with the non-medical issues that can result from cancer, such as financial problems, housing (when treatments must be taken at a facility away from home), and child care.

orchiectomy: surgery to remove the testicles; castration.

overflow incontinence: needing to get up often during the night to urinate, taking a long time to urinate and have a dribbling stream with little force. Overflow incontinence is usually due to blockage or narrowing of the bladder outlet, either from cancer or scar tissue.

p53: one of the tumor suppressor genes. Changes in this and similar genes may be responsible for making some prostate cancers more likely to grow and spread more rapidly than others.

PAP: *see* prostatic acid phosphatase.

PIN: *see* prostatic intraepithelial neoplasia.

PSA: *see* prostate-specific antigen.

palliative treatment: therapy that relieves symptoms, such as pain or blockage of urine flow, but is not expected to cure the cancer. Its main purpose is to improve the patient's quality of life.

pathologist: a doctor who specializes in diagnosis and classification of diseases by lab tests such as examining tissue and cells under a microscope. The pathologist determines whether a tumor is benign or cancerous, and, if cancerous, the exact cell type and grade.

pelvic lymph node dissection: removal of the lymph nodes in the pelvis.

pelvic nodes: pelvic lymph nodes; the lymph nodes, located within the pelvis, to which prostate cancer is most likely to spread. These nodes are often removed and examined for cancer (pelvic lymph node dissection) prior to radical prostatectomy.

pelvis: the part of the skeleton that forms a ring of bones in the lower trunk and that supports the spine and legs. Cancer may spread (metastasize) to these bones. Pelvis is also used to refer to the general region of the lower trunk surrounded by these bones.

penile implant: artificial device placed in the penis during surgery to restore erections.

penis: the male organ of copulation.

percent-free PSA: *see* free-PSA ratio.

perineal prostatectomy: an operation in which the prostate is removed through an incision in the skin between the scrotum and anus.

perineum: the area between the anus and the scrotum.

perineural invasion: invasion of cancer cells into areas around nerves in the prostate gland. This is sometimes reported by pathologists looking at prostatectomy specimens, but it is not thought to affect a man's prognosis.

peripheral zone: the largest part of the prostate, near the outer edges of the gland. It is where most prostate cancers occur.

permanent section: a method of preparation of tissue for microscopic examination. The tissue is soaked in formaldehyde, processed in various chemicals, surrounded by a block of wax, sliced very thin, attached to a microscope slide and stained. This usually takes 1–2 days. It provides a clear view of the sample so that the presence or absence of cancer can be determined.

phosphodiesterase inhibitors: drugs, such as sildenafil (Viagra), that can help men achieve an erection. Not all forms of impotence respond to these drugs, however.

platelet: a part of the blood that plugs up holes in blood vessels after an injury. Chemotherapy can cause a drop in the platelet count, a condition called thrombocytopenia that carries risk of excessive bleeding.

positive margin: *see* margin, surgical.

prevalence: a measure of the proportion of persons in the population with a particular disease at a given time. Compare with incidence.

primary site: the place where cancer begins. Primary cancer is named after the organ in which it starts. For example, cancer that starts in the prostate is always prostate cancer even if it spreads (metastasizes) to other organs such as bones or lymph nodes.

primary treatment: the first, and usually the most important, treatment.

prognosis: a prediction of the course of disease; the outlook for the chances of survival.

ProstaScint™ scan: like the bone scan, the ProstaScint scan uses low level radioactive material to find cancer that has spread beyond the prostate. But the radioactive material for the ProstaScint scan is attached to an antibody made in a lab to recognize and stick to a particular substance. In this case, the antibody sticks to prostate-specific membrane antigen (PSMA), a substance found only in normal and cancerous prostate cells. This test detects spread of prostate cancer to bone as well as lymph nodes and other organs, and that it can clearly distinguish prostate cancer from other cancers and benign disorders. It is most commonly used to look for cancer if the PSA level is elevated after treatment.

prostate: (note that there is no "r" in the second syllable) a gland found only in men. It is just below the bladder and in front of the rectum. The prostate makes a fluid that is part of semen. The tube that carries urine, the urethra, runs through the prostate.

prostate-specific antigen (PSA): a protein made by the prostate gland. Levels of PSA in the blood often go up in men with prostate cancer. The PSA test is used to help find prostate cancer as well as monitor the results of treatment.

prostatectomy: surgical removal of all or part of the prostate gland.

prostatic acid phosphatase (PAP): a blood test, like the PSA test, that may be done when looking for evidence of prostate cancer. Unlike the PSA test, the PAP test is not useful for prostate cancer screening.

prostatic intraepithelial neoplasia (PIN): a condition in which there are changes in the microscopic appearance of prostate epithelial cells. The condition is not cancer, but it may lead to the development of cancer.

prostatic urethra: the part of the urethra that runs through the prostate.

prostatitis: inflammation of the prostate, usually the result of an infection. Prostatitis is not cancer.

prosthesis: an artificial part used to replace or improve the function of a body part. A penile implant is an example of a prosthesis.

protocol: a formal outline or plan, such as a description of what treatments a patient will receive and exactly when each should be given. *See also* regimen.

proton: a radioactive particle used in some forms of radiation therapy. *See also* conformal proton beam radiation therapy.

PSA density (PSAD): PSAD is determined by dividing the PSA level by the prostate volume (its size as measured by transrectal ultrasound). A higher PSAD indicates greater likelihood of cancer.

PSA doubling time (PSADT): the amount of time it takes for the PSA level to double. This is sometimes useful in helping to determine if cancer is present or has recurred.

PSA velocity (PSAV): a measurement of how quickly the PSA level rises over a period of time. This has been suggested as a way to improve the accuracy of PSA testing. A higher PSAV indicates greater likelihood of cancer being present.

RT-PCR test: a very sensitive test for finding small numbers of prostate cancer cells in blood samples. It is still uncertain if or how the test should be used in considering treatment options.

rad: stands for "radiation absorbed dose," a measurement of the amount of radiation absorbed by tissues. The term rad is being replaced by cGy (centigray).

radiation oncologist: a doctor who specializes in using radiation to treat cancer.

radiation therapy: treatment with high-energy rays (such as x-rays) to kill or shrink cancer cells. The radiation may come from outside of the body (external radiation) or from radioactive materials placed directly in the tumor (brachytherapy or internal radiation). Radiation therapy may be used to reduce the size of a cancer before surgery, to destroy any remaining cancer cells after surgery, or as the main treatment. In advanced cancer cases, it may also be used as palliative treatment.

radiation proctitis: a possible side effect of radiation therapy, involving inflammation of the rectum and anus. Problems can include pain, bowel frequency, bowel urgency, bleeding, chronic burning, or rectal leakage.

radical prostatectomy: surgery to remove the entire prostate gland, the seminal vesicles and nearby tissue.

radiologist: a doctor with special training in diagnosis of diseases by interpreting x-rays and other types of diagnostic imaging studies; for example, CT and MRI scans.

radiopharmaceuticals: a group of drugs that include radioactive elements, such as strontium-89 or samarium-153, which are given intravenously (IV) to treat bone pain related to metastatic prostate cancer. *See also* strontium-89.

rectum: the lower part of the large intestine leading to the anus.

recurrence: cancer that has come back after treatment. Local recurrence means that the cancer has come back at the same place as the original cancer. Regional recurrence means that the cancer has come back after treatment in the lymph nodes near the primary site. Distant recurrence is when cancer metastasizes after treatment to distant organs or tissues (such as the lungs, liver, bone marrow, or brain).

red blood cells: blood cells that contain hemoglobin, the substance that carries oxygen to other tissues of the body.

refractory: no longer responsive to a certain therapy.

regimen: a strict, regulated plan (such as diet, exercise, or other activity) designed to reach certain goals. In cancer treatment, a plan to treat cancer. *See also* protocol.

regional involvement: the spread of cancer from its original site to nearby areas such as lymph nodes, but not to distant sites.

regression: reduction of the size of the tumor or the extent of the cancer.

rehabilitation: activities to help a person adjust, heal, and return to as full and productive a life as possible after injury or illness. This may involve physical restoration (such as the use of prostheses, exercises, and physical therapy), counseling, and emotional support.

relapse: reappearance of cancer after a disease-free period. *See also* recurrence.

relative five-year survival rate: the percentage of people with a certain cancer who have not died from it within 5 years. This number is different from the five-year survival rate in that it does not include people who have died from unrelated causes. Relative survival rates are important for prostate cancer because many men with it are older and may die from other health problems.

remission: complete or partial disappearance of the signs and symptoms of cancer in response to treatment; the period during which a disease is under control. A remission may not be a cure.

resectoscope: instrument used in transurethral resection of the prostate (TURP), allowing the surgeon direct inspection of the prostatic urethra and adjacent prostatic tissue.

response: outcome derived from treatment or reaction to a drug or any other therapy.

retention: *see* urinary retention.

retrograde ejaculation: a condition, often occurring after radiation, radical prostatectomy, or TURP, in which orgasm causes semen to enter the bladder, as opposed to exiting the body through the penis. Also known as a dry orgasm.

retropubic: behind the pubic bone; a surgical approach to the prostate through an incision in the lower abdomen (retropubic prostatectomy).

risk factor: anything that affects a person's chance of getting a disease such as cancer. Different cancers have different risk factors. For example, unprotected exposure to strong sunlight is a risk factor for skin cancer; smoking is a risk factor for lung, mouth, larynx, and other cancers. Some risk factors, such as smoking, can be controlled. Others, like a person's age, can't be changed.

saw palmetto: an herbal extract from the berries of the saw palmetto tree that is sometimes used to reduce symptoms of benign prostatic hyperplasia (BPH). It is not a proven treatment for prostate cancer.

screening: the search for disease, such as cancer, in people without symptoms. For example, screening measures for prostate cancer include digital rectal examination and the PSA blood test. Screening may refer to coordinated programs in large populations.

scrotum: the pouch of skin that holds the testicles.

selenium: a trace mineral that may play a role in reducing the risk of developing prostate cancer. Studies are now underway to determine if this is the case.

semen: fluid released during orgasm; it contains sperm and seminal fluid.

seminal vesicles: glands at the base of the bladder and next to the prostate that release fluid into the semen during orgasm. Cancer that spreads beyond the prostate gland may invade the seminal vesicles.

sextant biopsy: a biopsy of the prostate in which six core biopsy samples are taken, one each from the top, middle and bottom of each side of the prostate.

side effects: unwanted effects of treatment, such as hair loss caused by chemotherapy and fatigue caused by radiation therapy.

sign: an observable physical change caused by an illness. Compare to symptom.

simulation: a process involving special x-ray pictures that are used to plan radiation treatment so that the area to be treated is precisely located and marked for treatment.

sphincter, urethral: the muscle that squeezes the urethra shut and provides urinary control.

spinal cord compression: any process that results in pressure on the spinal cord, the spinal nerve trunks, or both; can occur when prostate cancer spreads to the spine.

staging: the process of finding out whether cancer has spread and if so, how far. There is more than one system for staging. The TNM system, which is used most often, gives three key pieces of information:

> **T** refers to the size of the **t**umor
>
> **N** describes how far the cancer has spread to nearby lymph **n**odes
>
> **M** tells whether the cancer has **m**etastasized (spread) to other organs of the body

Letters or numbers after the T, N, and M give more details about each of these factors. To make this information clearer, the TNM descriptions can be grouped together into a simpler set of stages, labeled with Roman numerals (usually from I to IV). In general, the lower the number, the less the cancer has spread. A higher number means a more serious cancer.

The two types of staging are:

> **clinical staging:** an estimate of the extent of cancer based on physical exam, biopsy results, and imaging tests.
>
> **pathologic staging:** an estimate of the extent of cancer by direct study of tissue removed during surgery.

standard therapy: the most commonly used and most widely accepted form of treatment; *see* therapy

stress incontinence: passing a small amount of urine when coughing, laughing, sneezing, or exercising.

stricture, urethral: a narrowing of the urethra due to scar tissue that blocks flow of urine and can result in overflow incontinence. This can be treated by surgically removing the scar tissue and stretching the urethra.

strontium-89: a radioactive substance that is used for treatment of bone pain due to metastatic prostate cancer. It is injected into a vein and is attracted to areas of bone containing metastatic cancer. The radiation given off by the strontium-89 kills the cancer cells, and relieves the pain caused by bone metastases.

survival rate: *see* five-year survival rate.

symptom: a change in the body caused by an illness, as described by the person experiencing it. Compare to sign.

TNM: *see* staging.

TRUS: *see* transrectal ultrasound.

TURP: *see* transurethral resection of the prostate.

testicles: the male reproductive glands found in the scrotum. The testicles (or testes) produce sperm and the male hormone testosterone.

testosterone: the main male hormone, made primarily in the testicles. It stimulates blood flow, growth in certain tissues, and the secondary sexual characteristics. In men with prostate cancer, it can also encourage growth of the tumor.

therapy: any of the measures taken to treat a disease. *See also* standard therapy, alternative therapy, complementary therapy, and unproven therapy.

three-dimensional conformal radiation therapy (3DCRT): this treatment uses sophisticated computers to very precisely map the location of the cancer within the prostate. The patient is fitted with a plastic mold resembling a body cast to keep him still so that the radiation can be more accurately aimed. Radiation beams are then aimed from several directions. This reduces the effects on normal tissues and may allow higher doses of radiation to be used.

tissue: a group of cells united to perform a particular function in the body.

total androgen blockade: *see* combination hormone therapy.

transition zone: innermost area of the prostate, surrounding the urethra. This is where benign prostatic hyperplasia (BPH) develops.

transrectal ultrasound (TRUS): an imaging test in which a probe inserted into the rectum gives off sound waves to create a picture of the prostate on a screen to help detect or find the location of tumors.

transurethral resection of the prostate (TURP): an operation that involves removing a part of the prostate gland that surrounds the urethra (the tube through which urine exits the bladder). The procedure is used for some men with prostate cancer who cannot have a radical prostatectomy because of advanced age or other serious illnesses. This operation can be used to relieve symptoms caused by a tumor, but it is not expected to cure this disease or remove all of the cancer. TURP is used more often to relieve symptoms of benign prostatic hyperplasia (BPH).

tumor: an abnormal lump or mass of tissue. Tumors can be benign (not cancerous) or malignant (cancerous).

tumor suppressor genes: genes that slow down cell division or cause cells to die at the appropriate time. Changes that inactivate these genes can lead to too much cell growth and development of cancer.

tumor volume: measure of the amount of cancer present.

unproven therapy: any therapy that has not been scientifically tested and approved.

ureters: tubes carrying urine from each kidney to the bladder.

urethra: the tube that carries urine from the bladder outside the body. In women, this tube is fairly short; in men it is longer, passing through the prostate and out through the penis, and it also carries the semen.

urge incontinence: a sudden and uncontrollable urge to pass urine. This problem occurs when the bladder becomes too sensitive to stretching by urine accumulation.

urgency: feeling that you need to urinate right away.

urinary retention: inability to empty the bladder; inability to urinate.

urodynamic study: test to evaluate function of the bladder muscle and sphincters.

urologist: a doctor who specializes in treating problems of the urinary tract in men and women, and of the genital area in men.

vacuum pump: a device that creates an erection by drawing blood into the penis; a ring placed at the base of the penis traps the blood and sustains the erection.

vas deferens: one of two muscular tubes that carry sperm from the testicles to the urethra.

vasectomy: surgery in which a segment of each vas deferens is removed to prevent release of sperm and thus provide contraception.

vitamin E: an antioxidant vitamin that may help prevent prostate cancer.

watchful waiting: a form of management of prostate cancer in which it is closely monitored (usually with PSA blood tests and digital rectal exams) instead of active treatment such as surgery or radiation therapy. This may be a reasonable choice for older men with small tumors that might grow very slowly. If the situation changes, active treatment can be started. Also known as expectant management.

white blood cells: cells that help defend the body against infections. There are several types of white blood cells. Certain cancer treatments such as chemotherapy can reduce the number of these cells and make a person more likely to get infections.

Whitmore-Jewett staging system: classification system for prostate cancer using the categories A, B, C, or D. It has largely been replaced by the TNM system. It can, however, be translated into the TNM system, or the doctor can explain how this staging system will determine treatment options.

x-ray: a form of radiation that can be used at low levels to produce an image of the body on film or at high levels to destroy cancer cells.

Index